Praise for *The Microbiome Solution*

"I whole-heartedly agree with Dr. Chutkan that there is a rising epidemic of vague symptoms often attributable to a damaged microbiome, from bloating and food intolerances to brain fog and weight-loss resistance. Her mantra 'Live dirty, eat clean!' is a scientifically-sound solution. Try her simple program—and get ready to feel the changes immediately. It's the proven way to build up our 'good bugs' and keep your body strong and vibrant, ready to fight illness and disease. It's something we can all do, each and every day. You will truly transform your health!"

—SARA GOTTFRIED, MD, author of the *New York Times* bestsellers *The Hormone Cure* and *The Hormone Reset Diet*

"We are truly in the middle of an epidemic—through our diet and our lifestyle we are unwittingly destroying the good bacteria in our bodies, the crucial allies we need to arm us against disease. In this life-changing book, Robynne Chutkan gives you simple, foolproof guidance to repair this vital ecosystem and bring you optimal health every day. Read this important book and discover the small changes that can make a huge impact."

—FRANK LIPMAN, MD, founder of Eleven Eleven Wellness Center and author of the *New York Times* bestseller *The New Health Rules*

"*The Microbiome Solution* is the medicine we all need to truly flourish."

—CHRISTIANE NORTHRUP, MD, author of the *New York Times* bestsellers *Goddesses Never Age*; *Women's Bodies, Women's Wisdom*; and *The Wisdom of Menopause*

"The exciting research on the microbiome has the promise to help many take charge of their health and reverse chronic ailments. But what is so groundbreaking about this book is that it shows you how to put these scientific breakthroughs into practice, step-by-step. With Dr. Robynne Chutkan as your guide, you'll understand how overuse of antibiotics, the standard Western diet, and a super-clean lifestyle starve your microbiome, and learn the essential tools to attain sustainable good health. This book is empowering, and indispensable for anyone trying to get or stay well."

—TERRY WAHLS, MD, author of *The Wahls Protocol*

"We live in symbiosis with trillions of bacteria that play a crucial role in determining our health and vitality. *The Microbiome Solution* is an eye-opening account of how supersanitation, antibiotic overuse, and the Western diet collaborate to promote chronic disease by disrupting the gut microbiome's ecological harmony and balance. Dr. Chutkan, a leading integrative gastroenterologist, presents a trailblazing program to heal your body from the inside-out by getting dirty and eating clean. Read this marvelous book and transform your health . . . one gut microbe at a time."

—GERARD E. MULLIN, MD, associate professor of medicine at The Johns Hopkins University School of Medicine and author of *The Gut Balance Revolution*

the
MICROBIOME
SOLUTION

the MICROBIOME SOLUTION

A RADICAL NEW WAY TO HEAL YOUR BODY FROM THE INSIDE OUT

Robynne Chutkan, MD, FASGE

AVERY
an imprint of Penguin Random House
New York

AVERY

an imprint of Penguin Random House LLC
375 Hudson Street
New York, New York 10014

First hardcover edition, August 2015
First trade paperback edition, August 2016
Copyright © 2015 by Robynne Chutkan

Most Avery books are available at special quantity discounts for bulk purchase for sales promotions, premiums, fund-raising, and educational needs. Special books or book excerpts also can be created to fit specific needs. For details, write SpecialMarkets@penguinrandomhouse.com.

Recipes courtesy of Elise Museles of Kale and Chocolate (www.kaleandchocolate.com). Reprinted with permission.

The Library of Congress has catalogued the hardcover edition as follows:

Chutkan, Robynne.
The microbiome solution : a radical new way to heal your body
from the inside out / Robynne Chutkan MD, FASGE.
p.   cm.
ISBN 978-1-58333-576-5
1. Gastrointestinal system—Diseases—Diet therapy.
2. Women—Health and hygiene—Popular works.   I. Title.
RC816.C484   2015   2015015884
616.3'30654—dc23

ISBN 978-0-399-57350-7 (paperback)

Printed in the United States of America
9   10   8

BOOK DESIGN BY TANYA MAIBORODA

To my parents, Winston and Noelle—
Thanks for a dirty childhood

Eat a peck of dirt before you die.

Contents

part 4 • Recipes

Acknowledgments

I am indebted to the many wonderful patients I've had the privilege of caring for who have taught me so much over the last two decades.

My husband, Eric, and daughter, Sydney, have been enthusiastic and joyful participants in our ongoing Live Dirty, Eat Clean experiment. I am so grateful to you both.

And a heartfelt thank-you to my wonderful team at Avery—Lucia Watson, Gigi Campo, Megan Newman, Anne Kosmoski, and to Toni Sciarra Poynter and Howard Yoon. You make writing books a lot of fun.

Introduction:
Live Dirty, Eat Clean

M Y HUSBAND ISN'T completely on board with my plan to sell our house in the city, move to a farm, raise animals, and grow our own food. But since much of what's available in the supermarket is full of chemicals and devoid of any real nutrients, taking control of what we eat and making sure it comes from nature, not a factory, strikes me as a good idea. I'm fortunate to live in Washington, D.C., where farmers' markets and community supported agriculture (CSA) shares are plentiful, so moving to an actual farm may seem a little extreme. My real motivation is that I want my daughter to grow up dirty, literally—as in easy on the soap and shampoo, heavy on the mucky animal chores. I shared her saga of antibiotic misadventure in my first book, *Gutbliss*. Since then, I've seen hundreds of patients with stories similar to hers, and I've become even more convinced that damage to the microbiome—the trillions of organisms that call our digestive tract home—is at the root of many of our current health problems. Figuring out how to undo that damage and "rewild" ourselves has become a focus of my medical practice and a personal journey in our household. Living a little dirtier and eating a little cleaner is definitely part of the fix.

Unwilding Ourselves

Our ancestors had a symbiotic relationship with their microbes that evolved over millions of years and served them well. They were benevolent hosts to a dense jungle of microscopic creatures, including worms and other parasites that actually contributed to their health. Large predators and the absence of food were their main threats, not the hundreds of diseases that afflict us today. The irony is that as we've "unwilded" our bodies and our environment in an effort to become healthier, we've actually become a lot sicker in some important ways.

Urbanization and modern medicine have undoubtedly improved our lives, but they've also introduced practices—overuse of antibiotics, chlorination of the water supply, processed foods full of chemicals and hormones, microbe-depleting pesticides, increasing rates of Cesarean sections—that have ravaged our microbiome, diminishing the total number of organisms as well as the diversity of species. The result is an increase in a wide range of modern plagues, including asthma, allergies, autoimmune diseases, diabetes, obesity, cancer, irritable bowel syndrome, anxiety, and heart disease. The rise of these diseases is inextricably intertwined with the full-on assault on our microbiome resulting from our super-sanitized lifestyle.

A decade ago, who knew that every antibiotic dispensed during cold and flu season was potentially bringing us one step closer to a diagnosis of Crohn's disease, or making us fatter? None of us doing the prescribing realized that we might be paving the way to real illness in our well-meaning attempts to cure the sniffles. The prevailing wisdom was—and to some extent still is—that germs are bad and we should get rid of them, and antibiotics are good and we should use them. And use them we have: the average American child will receive more than a dozen courses of antibiotics before reaching college, primarily for minor illnesses that require no treatment at all. Despite the tremendous amount of research in the last few years connecting the dots, many physicians and their patients remain in the dark, blaming each manifestation of microbial discord on bad luck or bad genes, never questioning or understanding the root cause.

Less Is Often More

My own understanding came only after my daughter was treated with antibiotics at birth and throughout infancy, setting off a series of events that, a decade later, continue to affect her health. I had been trained at world-class institutions and practiced gastroenterology at a leading teaching hospital, but, like most physicians, I had no idea that the antibiotics I thought were so helpful were actually creating illness by decimating her microbiome at a time when it was most vulnerable, making her more susceptible to infection and inflammation. I wish I had known then what I know now and what I continue to learn every day: that illness is often the result of a decreased, not increased, bacterial load, and that less is sometimes more when it comes to medical intervention.

Rehab for Your Microbiome

Every day in my gastroenterology practice I see patients with the telltale signs of a disordered microbiome: bloating, leaky gut, irritable bowel, gluten intolerance, Crohn's disease, ulcerative colitis, eczema, thyroid disorders, weight problems, fatigue, and brain fog. It's a veritable epidemic of "missing microbes," as infectious disease specialist Martin Blaser, MD, describes it. The symptoms vary, but the history doesn't: overzealous use of antibiotics, often accompanied by a highly processed Western diet low in indigestible plant fiber—the preferred food of gut bacteria.

Repopulating the microbiome can be a challenging process, but the good news is that most people do get better. Your microbes are constantly changing and evolving, and even if they've been severely damaged by medications, infection, or diet, paying attention to what you put in and on your body can yield huge improvements. The microbiome you have today isn't the one you were born with, nor is it the one you'll have next year or even next week. It's highly dynamic, constantly changing and adjusting in response to your internal and external environment.

In medical school, I was taught how to eradicate people's germs. A quarter-century later, I'm teaching my patients how to restore theirs: which foods to eat, how to care for their bodies and their homes without stripping away their microbes, what questions to ask when their doctor recommends an antibiotic, and whether a probiotic or even a stool transplant might be of benefit. These, I believe, are the new and essential survival skills for thriving in our super-clean era. You'll find them all in the Live Dirty, Eat Clean Plan at the end of this book.

When Dirty Children Grow into Clean Adults—My Rewilding Journey

I spent my early childhood in the tropics, eating food from my grandfather's farm grown in rich soil fertilized by a herd of goats (which we sometimes also ate) instead of chemicals. We lived in the hilly suburbs and roamed around outside with our dog after school, exploring gullies, picking mangoes and oranges from the fruit trees in our backyard, and acquiring the occasional case of pinworm as a result of our barefoot explorations. In our household there was lots of attention paid to schoolwork and athletics, but shoes, showers, and shampoos were more or less optional. My father was an orthopedic surgeon whose great fear was that his children would grow up to be hypochondriacs, so his medical advice for whatever ailed us—from the flu to a sprained ankle—was always the same: go lie down and you'll feel better in the morning. We were vaccinated for the big stuff (polio and smallpox) but didn't sweat the small stuff (whooping cough and chicken pox). My daughter had more visits to the doctor before she was in preschool than I've had in my entire lifetime.

So, despite my dirty childhood filled with organic, homegrown food, protective parasites, lots of time outdoors, and limited contact with an overzealous medical system, how did I end up in adulthood with not one but three manifestations of microbial discord: eczema, rosacea, and yeast overgrowth? It took a while. I managed to weather potent microbial disruptors like the antibiotics prescribed in college for acne and twenty years of birth control pills (we'll talk about this more in Chapter 5) with no ill effects. But as life got more complicated, unrelenting stress and the cookies, cakes, and candy I consumed to combat it were my ultimate undoing. A Western diet high in sugar and fat promotes growth of the wrong types of bacteria in your gut, and a lifestyle that leaves literally no time to go outside and smell the roses can be the straw that breaks the camel's back, particularly if you have additional risk factors, as I did, such as significant antibiotic use.

Disease Begins in Your Microbiome

My firsthand experience with how poor nutrition and stress can unmask the effects of a damaged microbiome and lead to a multitude of symptoms is representative of what most of the patients I see in my office have experienced: a decline in overall well-being characterized by seemingly unrelated conditions that appear out of nowhere, leaving them scratching their head and wondering what's going on.

Microbial disruptors are everywhere—in the food we eat, the water we drink, the products we use, and the medications we take—and the clinical manifestations of a disrupted microbiome are varied and show up in people of all ages and stages. Chances are there's someone in your family with asthma, allergies, eczema, thyroiditis, diabetes, arthritis, or any of the many disorders that we're now discovering have the same root cause. A damaged microbiome isn't the only reason people develop these conditions, but it's often a major contributor that interacts with genetic and environmental factors to create a perfect storm of disease.

That's why it's more important than ever to understand the complex and critical role bacteria play in our health, so that if and when yours is compromised, you can connect the dots and start to heal yourself.

The solutions you'll find in this book are based on clinical trials in our own patient population at the Digestive Center for Women, data from other scientific studies, published papers, trial and error, anecdote, patient testimonials about what's worked for them, and careful observations accrued over almost two decades of taking care of people with all kinds of bacterial imbalance—from serious autoimmune illnesses such as Crohn's disease and ulcerative colitis to complaints of gas and bloating. They're also based on my own journey of exploration and healing necessitated by my health challenges.

The new paradigm of bacteria as friend rather than foe is at the heart of a revolution in health care that's forcing us to reexamine how we live, as well as our medical practices, with new microscopic eyes, and to consider how modern life and our everyday choices affect the life of our microbes—and how our microbes in turn affect us. What has become very clear is that our individual and collective health depends on it. My sincere hope is that this book will provide you with the microbiome solution that will help you reclaim your health and vitality and set you on the path to a dirtier and disease-free life.

See you on the farm!

part 1

GETTING TO KNOW YOUR GUT BACTERIA

||||||||||||||||||||||||||||||||||||||||||||

CHAPTER 1

The Zoo Inside You

OUR MICROBES ARE intimately involved in every aspect of our health—from ensuring our digestive well-being to influencing our likelihood of being obese and our risk of developing cancer or diabetes. They even play a role in our brain chemistry and mental health, affecting our moods, our emotions, and our personalities. We are, it seems, single individuals comprised of multiple living, breathing, moving parts. The more we learn about this fascinating microscopic community, the clearer it becomes that our fate is inextricably tied to theirs, making it essential that we learn more about where our microbes come from, what they do, and why we literally can't live without them.

Meet Your Microbiome

The microbiome refers to all of the organisms that live in or on your body: all of the bacteria, viruses, fungi, protozoa, and helminths (worms, for those of us who have them), as well as all of their genes. A staggering hundred trillion microbes that include thousands of different species inhabit your nooks and crannies—with more than a billion bacteria in *just one drop* of fluid in your colon alone.

Your unique microbial footprint develops over your lifetime, and it reflects everything about you: your parents' health, how and where you were born, what you've eaten (including whether your first sips were breast milk or formula), where you've lived, your occupation, personal hygiene, past infections, exposure to chemicals and toxins, medications, hormone levels, and even your emotions (stress can have a profound effect on the microbiome). The end result is a microbial mix so distinctive from person to person that yours is a more accurate identifier of you than your own DNA.

We've known about the microbiome since the 1600s, when Antoni van Leeuwenhoek first looked at his own dental plaque under the microscope and described "little living animalcules, very prettily a-moving." But it's taken us a few centuries to figure out that these fellow travelers might actually be helping rather than hindering us, with a specific purpose that's very much aligned with our own survival. The overwhelming majority of our microbes aren't germs that cause disease. Quite the contrary—they're an essential part of our ecosystem and play a vital role in keeping us healthy.

How do we get from germ-free fetus to living, breathing petri dish, colonized with trillions of bacteria? Let's start at the cradle and work our way toward the grave, to find out exactly how our microbiome evolves and the crucial role it plays at every stage in our development.

Pregnancy

Long before we enter the world, our mother's microbiome starts to prepare for our arrival. One of the most dramatic changes happens in her vagina. During pregnancy, cells in the vaginal lining ramp up production of a carbohydrate called glycogen, sending glycogen-loving *Lactobacillus* bacteria into a feeding frenzy and increasing their numbers. *Lactobacilli* convert lactose and other sugars to lactic acid, creating an acidic, unfriendly environment that helps to protect the growing fetus from potential invaders.

Bacteria don't just protect us from undesirable germs that can enter via the vagina; they also nurture us. In the third trimester of pregnancy, *Proteobacteria* and *Actinobacteria* species increase in number and cause a corresponding rise in the mother's blood sugar and weight gain in her breasts, with the specific goal of ensuring adequate growth and breast milk for the baby. Transplanting gut bacteria from late-trimester pregnant women into nonpregnant mice produces identical changes in the mice—confirming that the transformation is indeed mediated by gut bacteria, not hormones.

In addition to our founding species of bacteria, we also receive protective antibodies from our mother through the placenta. Armed with these antibodies and our own few but plucky microbial soldiers, we're ready to make our entrance into the world. But exactly how we enter isn't just a matter of convenience; it has significant microbial repercussions that continue to affect our health well into adulthood.

Birth

During a normal delivery, the baby's head turns to face the mother's rectum as it crowns and exits the birth canal. This turning brings the baby's nose and mouth into direct contact with her vaginal and rectal contents. What better way to get inoculated with a good dose of bacteria than to come face-to-tush with the source? A study published in *Proceedings of the National Academy of Sciences* showed that babies born vaginally are colonized with *Lactobacillus* species and other "good bacteria," while babies born by C-section tend to have more common hospital "bad bacteria" like *Staphylococcus* that are associated with illness and infection.

This brief act of swallowing a mouthful of our mother's microbes as we enter the world confers unbelievably important benefits. It turns out that exposure to bacteria is a critical early step in the development of our immune system. C-sections bypass this crucial event and are associated with higher rates of asthma, allergies, obesity, type 1 diabetes, and other autoimmune conditions. I'll explain the importance of early microbial exposure in detail in Chapter 3, and the modern plagues that are a result of not having enough of it.

Breast-feeding

Human milk oligosaccharides (HMOs) are the third-most common ingredient in breast milk, despite the fact that they're completely indigestible by infants. HMOs are indigestible because they're not there to feed the baby. They're there to feed the baby's bacteria—specifically, *Bifidobacterium*, present in high numbers in breast-fed infants. *Bifidobacterium* repels *Staphylococcus* and other harmful microbes on the mother's nipple, so it's an essential part of the baby's microbial arsenal. While *Bifidobacterium* gorges on HMOs, *Lactobacillus* in the newborn's gut breaks down sugars and the other digestible components of breast milk—an incredibly well-designed example of the symbiotic relationship between humans and microbes.

Breast-fed babies in the United States have an astounding 20 percent higher survival rate than their formula-fed peers. I'll discuss the worrisome trend of formula over breast milk in Chapter 7, where we examine the microbial implications of some of our modern practices.

Infancy

When we are babies, everything eventually ends up in our mouth. It's one of the ways we interact with our environment. It's also one of the ways our environment interacts with our microbiome, allowing bacteria from our home, our siblings, and even our pets to gain access to our gut and help train our immune system to distinguish friend from foe. Factors like family size, early nutrition, and the quality of our water supply have a profound effect on our blossoming microbiome.

Not surprisingly, as infants our microbiome most closely resembles that of other household members, especially our mothers. But it's a constantly changing and evolving mix, with lots of species diversity, and events like a fever, a dietary change, or a course of antibiotics can have a major ripple effect. Within a few weeks after birth, bacteria in various parts of our body start to branch out and specialize, and within a few months, the number of species starts to rise, increasing from about a hundred in infancy to a thousand or more by adulthood.

Childhood to Adulthood

By age three our microbiome is almost fully formed and is very similar to that of an adult, although major changes like puberty, the onset of menstruation, pregnancy, and menopause are associated with huge microbial shifts. Some of the physical changes associated with puberty, such as increased oil production that can lead to acne, or more pungent body odor under the arms and in the groin, are actually the result of changes in bacteria, as different species become more or less dominant.

By the time we become senior citizens, we've lost much of our bacterial diversity, and our microbiome starts to resemble that of others in our peer group. Shifts within various microbial populations continue to occur, but as we get older, our microbiome becomes more stable, tending to revert to its previously established baseline after events like an infection or a course of antibiotics.

Renewal

We start out in the womb with no microbes at all, and we eventually acquire trillions. What happens to all of those microbes when we die? Interestingly, the microbes aren't recycled. They die with us, and each subsequent generation goes through its own cycle of microbial rebirth, starting from scratch and working its way up to an incredibly well-stocked microbial kingdom, well adapted (let's hope) to the requirements of that generation.

Diversity of species is a vital part of maintaining a balanced ecosystem in the outside world, and it's also crucial in the microscopic world inside us. Unfortunately, modern life has made microbial depletion part of our legacy, with decreased diversity in each successive generation as a result of medications, our overprocessed diet, and our supersanitized lifestyle. Americans today have only about two-thirds as many bacterial species as native tribesmen in the Amazon who haven't been exposed to antibiotics. As we'll learn in the second part of this book, restoring those lost microbes takes real commitment.

While there is no perfect microbiome, some are clearly healthier than others, notwithstanding the incredible variation from one to the other. The Human Microbiome Project and other research efforts like it seek to establish what the "normal" human microbiome looks like today—an important endeavor, considering the rate at which our microbial landscape is changing. Companies like uBiome allow the citizen scientist to catalogue his or her own microscopic habitat, compare it to others, and reassess it as diet and habits change.

The human microbiome may well be the next big frontier in medicine, providing answers to why we get sick and novel solutions for how to heal ourselves. In the next chapter we'll learn more about what our gut bacteria actually do—besides make gas—and why they're so essential to our health and well-being.

CHAPTER 2

|||||||||||||||||||||||||||||||||||||||||||

Microbes: Your Worker Bees

THINK OF YOUR BODY as a factory. Organs like your lungs, kidneys, and liver represent the machinery that keeps production moving: extracting oxygen, filtering blood, removing toxins, synthesizing hormones, and performing all of the other complicated tasks that keep us alive. Some of the tasks are automated, but most of these assembly lines require constant monitoring, maintenance, and adjustment.

We house the machinery, but who operates it? How does a complex process like, for example, digestion, actually happen? Who helps break down the food and determines what gets absorbed versus what gets excreted? How do we distinguish between real infection and colonization with harmless bacteria? Who tells our immune system when to rally the troops and when to ignore benign interlopers that pose no threat?

Our microbes do! We've evolved over millions of years to host an incredible army of worker bee microbes that are gainfully employed assisting in all of our bodily functions. They produce substances our bodies require but can't make. They fight most of our battles for us. They even turn our genes on and off, activating those we need and dismantling those we don't. In exchange, we provide room and board.

Since we're their host and they rely on us for their survival, most of our microbes are invested in our well-being, although under certain circumstances they can turn on us and cause bad things to happen such as infection or even cancer. We can categorize our microscopic roommates into three main groups:

1. Commensal bacteria that cohabit peacefully with us
2. Symbiotic organisms (sometimes called mutualists) that help keep us healthy
3. Pathogens (also known as opportunistic flora) that can do us harm

It's a Jungle in There

Most human bacteria fall within four general phyla, or families: *Actinobacteria*, *Firmicutes*, *Proteobacteria*, and *Bacteroidetes*—each one consisting of many different species. Different parts of the body have different microbial communities based on variations in things like oxy-

---

TABLE 2–1 • Predominant Bacteria Present in Humans

Location	Bacteria
Skin	*Staphylococci, Corynebacteria*
Nose	*Staphylococci, Corynebacteria*
Mouth	*Streptococci, Lactobacilli*
Throat	*Streptococci, Neisseria*
Stomach	*Helicobacter pylori*
Small intestine	*Bifidobacteria, Enterococci*
Colon	*Bacteroides, Enterococci, Clostridia*
Urinary tract	*Staphylococci, Corynebacteria*
Vagina	*Lactic acid bacteria*

gen content, moisture, and blood flow. Anaerobic species that don't require oxygen predominate in the gut; *Staphylococci* thrive on the skin; and the same *Streptococci* used to make Swiss cheese inhabit the mouth and upper airway. There are pathogenic (i.e., harmful) forms of all of these bacteria, but the ones that reside with us on a daily basis are mostly harmless, particularly when kept in check by adequate amounts of their symbiotic cousins.

An enterotype is a classification based on ecosystems in the gut, and a way to stratify people based on the relative abundance of different species. In 2011, researcher Peer Bork described three specific enterotypes in humans: high levels of *Bacteroides* characterize type 1; type 2 has few *Bacteroides* and lots of *Prevotella*; and type 3 has high levels of *Ruminococcus*. Different enterotypes don't seem to be influenced by age, gender, or nationality, but they are profoundly affected by long-term diet. A Western diet high in protein and animal fat is associated with *Bacteroides* (type 1), while *Prevotella* species (type 2) dominate in those who consume more carbohydrates, especially fiber. Different enterotypes are associated with predisposition to particular disease states, such as obesity and inflammation, confirming that what you eat is a powerful influencer of your overall health. In the future, we may be able to prescribe enterotype-specific diets and probiotics designed for maximal efficacy based on the abundance of various species.

What Do Gut Bacteria Do?

Symbiotic organisms—the quintessential good bacteria—have lots of important jobs. They help us digest food, maintain the integrity of our gut lining (part of the epithelial barrier that keeps bowel contents separate from the rest of the body), crowd out harmful bacteria, and train our immune system to distinguish between friend and foe. They also convert sugars into short-chain fatty acids (SCFAs) that intestinal cells use for energy, and they synthesize many of the enzymes, vitamins, and hormones that we can't make on our own. Food can't be properly broken down and its constituent parts can't be fully absorbed without these essential gut bacteria, which means that even if you're eating a super-healthy diet, if you don't have enough of them, you may not be able to absorb and assimilate all of the vitamins and nutrients in your food.

Most of the bacteria in your gut are anaerobic, meaning that they thrive in areas with little or no oxygen. As you travel from the top to the bottom of the intestines, the amount of bacteria increases, so the stomach and small intestine have a lot less than the colon. Some bacterial species set up shop in the intestinal lining, while others just pass through, sometimes reproducing while in transit before being excreted in the stool.

TABLE 2–2 • What Do Your Gut Bacteria Do?

- Convert sugars to short-chain fatty acids (SCFAs) for energy
- Crowd out pathogens
- Digest food
- Help your body absorb nutrients such as calcium and iron
- Keep pH balanced
- Maintain the integrity of the gut lining
- Metabolize drugs
- Modulate genes
- Neutralize cancer-causing compounds
- Produce digestive enzymes
- Synthesize B-complex vitamins (thiamine, folate, pyridoxine)
- Synthesize fat-soluble vitamins (vitamin K)
- Synthesize hormones
- Train the immune system to distinguish friend from foe

Immune Regulation

Digestion isn't the only process that relies on the presence of gut bacteria. Exposure to lots of different microbes—both good and bad—is essential for priming and training your immune system, so that later on it's able to distinguish between harmless organisms that it should ignore and dangerous pathogens that it needs to respond to. In Chapter 7 we'll find out what happens when we super-sanitize our environment and miss out on that crucial early microbial exposure.

Gene Modulation

We have about twenty-three thousand human genes and eight million microbial ones. Results from large-scale human microbiome studies suggest that genes from gut bacteria play an important role. They provide instructions for essential functions like carbohydrate metabolism and enzymatic detoxification—instructions that are missing from our own human genome. Bacteria also help determine which diseases are expressed, turning various human genes on and off in response to the body's internal milieu, which can influence whether or not a disease that you're genetically predisposed to actually develops. Modulation of our genes by bacteria may explain why inherited diseases don't always afflict family members equally—even in identical twins, who have the same genes but different microbes.

You're Only as Healthy as Your Gut Bacteria

Ever notice how some people never get sick when everyone else has the flu? They were probably exposed to the same virulent virus, but because they have a healthier microbiome populated with more essential microbes, they're able to crowd out the pathogens and stay healthy. Antibiotics can actually make you *more* susceptible to infection because they deplete essential bacterial species that can fight off viruses and dangerous bacteria. A recent study injected a bacterial protein into mice suffering from Rotavirus—a diarrheal illness that kills half a million children each year—and successfully halted the infection. The same protein also showed efficacy against other viruses, including influenza, demonstrating the important role bacteria play in protecting against viral infection.

Microbial health is one of the factors that determines who survives potentially deadly viruses. The very young, whose microbiome is still developing, and the very old, who have fewer microbial species and less diversity, tend to be the most vulnerable. Overzealous antibiotic use also puts you at risk by stripping out the good microbes along with the bad. Of course, additional variables like coexisting medical problems and how well nourished you are play a role, too, but those factors are also tied to the health of your microbiome, so having enough good bacteria looms large as a way to protect yourself from acute as well as chronic illness.

Allison is a patient I see for chronic constipation and bloating. While her gastrointestinal (GI) symptoms have improved a lot with adding more fiber to her diet, she continues to be plagued by chronic sinus infections. Every time I see her she's either on an antibiotic or just finished taking one. The more antibiotics she takes, the more sinus infections she seems to get. We'll take an in-depth look at how heavy antibiotic use can compromise your microbiome in Chapter 4, "Pharmageddon and the Antibiotic Paradox."

Recognizing that infection is frequently a result of bacterial imbalance as opposed to infestation with any one particular bad bug helps us to be more judicious in our approach to treatment. We all have organisms within us whose growth, if left unchecked, can reach problematic proportions. The solution isn't to embark on a search-and-destroy antimicrobial mission, devastating our essential bacteria along with the bad guys, but rather to repopulate and rebalance, adding good bacteria through dietary changes, microbe-friendly practices, prebiotic foods, and a well-chosen probiotic supplement. My Live Dirty, Eat Clean Plan will tell you exactly how to accomplish that, improving any health issues you have now and helping to safeguard against future illness.

The Nose Knows

Our different anatomical microbial communities have their own distinctive signature odors, based on what the various bacteria consume and the waste products they make. Morning breath is a great example of how shifting microbial populations are associated with a distinct change in odor. Most of us sleep with our mouth closed, breathing mostly through our nose. That leads to lower levels of oxygen in the mouth and an overnight increase in anaerobic bacteria, whose by-products give our breath a sour smell. People who have inflammation in their colon from Crohn's disease, ulcerative colitis, or acute infection also have significant shifts in the composition of their gut bacteria— changes that I can smell even before seeing when I insert the colonoscope to examine the colon.

Most animals can detect variations in the microbiome. They sniff each other for recognition, to tell whether females are in heat, and to detect fear in their prey. If we deigned to take a whiff, we'd notice lots of identifying features, too—who has smelly feet, eats a lot of meat, or is stressed out—it's all reflected in our microbiome. I smell my daughter all the time (much to her dismay), and as she approaches puberty, I'm noticing lots of changes. But mostly I just know what she smells like, the specific aroma that is unique to her and that I like to think I could recognize anywhere.

Growing a Good Gut Garden

As I've mentioned, there's incredible microbial variation from person to person, which makes it difficult to define exactly what the ideal microbiome looks (or smells) like. Our health depends on having the right balance, without any one species becoming unnaturally dominant or submissive, and with essential bacteria sufficiently represented.

Gut bacteria are influenced by all the factors I've already mentioned, like whether you were breast-fed, your age, your gender, your occupation, and where you live. But what you eat is emerging as the most influential factor, since bacteria follow the food. So rather than focusing on what you should be eating to lose weight, or to lower your cholesterol, or to avoid diabetes, you should really be asking yourself what you should be eating to grow a good gut garden, because disease is rare when gut bacteria are balanced, bountiful, and diverse.

The other essential step is recognizing what threatens your gut garden's growth. Being aware of the interlopers and inclement conditions that will reduce your victory garden to an overgrown or blighted plot is key. In the next part of this book we'll explore in detail how the microbiome gets messed up, and what you can do to preserve yours.

part 2

————————

MESSING UP THE MICROBIOME

CHAPTER 3

||||||||||||||||||||||||||||||||||||||||||||

The Hygiene Hypothesis
and Our Modern Plagues

MANY OF US were brought up to believe that it's better to be clean than dirty. But evidence is mounting to show that if you start from that premise, you will arrive at the wrong destination as far as human health is concerned. The microbial communities established in our bodies at birth, during infancy, and in early childhood mold our health as we grow and help determine whether or not we develop illness. The unwilding of our internal landscape has created health challenges we never anticipated and led to the emergence of a new breed of disease.

Microbes and Our Modern Plagues

In 1932, gastroenterologist Burrill Crohn, MD, and his colleagues at Mount Sinai Hospital published a paper describing fourteen patients who had peculiar findings in the small intestine at surgery that were unlike anything that had previously been seen. The abnormalities were in the end of the small intestine—an area known as the ileum—so they called the new disease terminal ileitis, although it would eventually come to be known as Crohn's disease.

Inflammatory bowel diseases (IBD), such as Crohn's disease and its sister condition, ulcerative colitis, are examples of autoimmune diseases. They represent a new breed of malady, sometimes referred to as modern plagues, which has emerged in the last century and includes conditions such as Hashimoto's thyroiditis, type 1 diabetes, lupus, multiple sclerosis (MS), rheumatoid arthritis, and eczema. Their hallmark, regardless of what organ they affect, is that the immune system wages war against the body's own healthy tissues, leading to chronic inflammation.

There are almost a hundred different types of autoimmune diseases. Chances are you or someone in your family suffers from one, since they affect about fifty million people in the United States alone. Dif-

TABLE 3-1 • Common Autoimmune Diseases

- Addison's disease
- Alopecia areata
- Ankylosing spondylitis
- Celiac disease
- Crohn's disease
- Dermatomyositis
- Diabetes (type 1)
- Eczema
- Eosinophilic esophagitis
- Graves' disease
- Hashimoto's thyroiditis
- Idiopathic thrombocytopenic purpura (ITP)
- Interstitial cystitis
- Juvenile arthritis
- Lupus (SLE)
- Multiple sclerosis (MS)
- Myasthenia gravis
- Polymyositis
- Primary biliary cirrhosis
- Primary sclerosing cholangitis
- Psoriasis
- Psoriatic arthritis
- Raynaud's phenomenon
- Rheumatoid arthritis
- Sarcoidosis
- Scleroderma
- Sjögren's syndrome
- Ulcerative colitis
- Urticaria
- Vasculitis
- Vitiligo

ferent autoimmune diseases frequently affect the same person, suggesting a common cause with varied manifestations rather than multiple distinct ailments. The million-dollar question is whether that common cause is an abnormal immune system overreacting to normal stimuli in the environment, or a normal immune system responding to an abnormal trigger.

Understanding the relationship between our immune system, our microbial environment, and our genes is critical to figuring out why people suffer from these diseases and how to heal them. Since most of our germs and more than half of our immune system are located in our gut, taking a closer look at Crohn's disease in the context of the microbiome may yield some valuable answers.

Guts, Germs, and Genes

Dr. Crohn was convinced that this new disease, which caused inflammation, weight loss, and diarrhea, was the result of a bacterial infection, although not everyone shared his view. At that time, Crohn's disease was most often diagnosed in people of Jewish heritage, and the prevailing wisdom was that Crohn's was a genetic rather than an infectious disease. The bacterium in question was *Mycobacterium avium subspecies paratuberculosis* (MAP). It was known to infect the same area of the ileum in cows and other ruminants, causing a Crohn's-like wasting diarrheal illness in these animals called Johne's disease (after the German veterinarian who described it in 1905).

In addition to the similarities in location and symptoms, there were two other compelling pieces of evidence in support of Dr. Crohn's theory that bacterial infection caused Crohn's disease. The first was that MAP had been isolated from the intestines of Crohn's patients at much higher rates than in the general public. The second was that because of its ability to survive pasteurization, MAP was detectable in various milk products, providing a plausible way for it to get from cows to humans. But what kept this from all fitting together nicely was that not everyone who had Crohn's disease had MAP. In fact, most Crohn's sufferers tested negative for MAP. So, after additional studies were unable to prove clear cause and effect, the idea that Crohn's was the result of a bacterial infection was mostly abandoned.

Almost a century later, we still don't know what causes autoimmune illnesses such as Crohn's, although there's been lots of speculation—from infections like measles, *E. coli*, and enterovirus to lifestyle factors like smoking and stress to common and seemingly benign practices like the use of toothpaste and refrigeration. In keeping with Dr. Crohn's initial theory, emerging evidence suggests that bacteria do indeed play a major role, but it may be their *absence* rather than their presence that leads to the diagnosis.

The Hygiene Hypothesis

In the late 1950s, Professor David Strachan, a lecturer at the London School of Hygiene and Tropical Medicine, embarked on an epidemiological study of hay fever and eczema in British children. These diseases had been steadily increasing since the turn of the century when large populations left the farm for the factory. The study followed seventeen thousand children from birth to adulthood, and the results revealed a startling and unexpected association: both conditions were far less common in large families with lots of early childhood infections from exposure to siblings. The highest rates of disease occurred in smaller family size with fewer runny-nosed microbial donors and in affluent households with loftier standards of personal hygiene. This finding was counter to everything we thought we knew about germs. Could exposure to more germs really be better for us? And could living a cleaner lifestyle be making us sicker?

Strachan's initial paper, titled "Hay Fever, Hygiene and Household Size," was published in the *British Medical Journal* in 1989 and laid the foundation for the "hygiene hypothesis," which challenged the idea of germs as something to be avoided and posited the importance of early microbial exposure for preventing disease later in life. In 2003 Graham Rook, MD, emeritus professor of medical microbiology and immunology at University College London, expanded on this concept with his "Old Friends" hypothesis, suggesting that a lack of exposure to ancient organisms like parasites that coevolved with our ancestors, not just the absence of relatively new germs like influenza, was responsible for the emergence of these modern plagues.

If we look at a map of the world today, one of the striking observations is that illnesses like Crohn's disease are common in more developed countries and rare in less developed ones. The hygiene hypothesis accounts for this uneven distribution by suggesting that *less* childhood exposure to bacteria and parasites in affluent societies like the United States and Europe actually *increases* susceptibility to disease by suppressing the natural development of the immune system.

This concept has also been linked to the rise of many of our chronic ailments: the obesity epidemic, deadly disorders like metabolic syndrome and heart disease, psychiatric conditions like depression, poorly understood afflictions like autism, and even some forms of cancer— and clinical studies have shown significant disturbances in the microbiome in all of them. We spend huge amounts of time making sure we're clean—scrubbing ourselves with harsh soaps, sanitizing our hands and environment with chemicals, and eliminating any trace of dirt from our homes and lives—but since the evidence suggests that germs may actually be essential for our well-being, it may be time to rethink our approach to cleanliness and hygiene.

In Praise of Dirt

We need interaction with dirt and germs to train our immune system in how to respond appropriately to stimuli in our environment—what to react to and what to ignore. An immune system that doesn't get up close and personal with enough germs early on is like a kid with over-protective parents, ill equipped to deal with problems when they inevitably happen. Inadequate exposure leads to defects in immune tolerance and a trigger-happy state of heightened activity where essential bacteria, proteins in food, and even parts of our own body (the digestive tract, in the case of IBD) are treated like the enemy and attacked.

While those living in poor countries with fewer modern conveniences are at higher risk of suffering the effects of natural disasters, poverty, and unemployment, from an autoimmune perspective there are some advantages, including much lower rates of Crohn's. Not surprisingly, as countries become more industrialized and their level of sanitation improves, the prevalence of IBD and what we might call other post–Industrial Revolution epidemics increases dramatically. We've seen examples of this in Asia and the Middle East, where clinics devoted to Crohn's have sprung up in the last decade in regions where the disease was previously nonexistent.

I certainly don't mean to romanticize poverty or suggest that economic growth and development are bad things, but it's worth pointing out that modern practices such as chlorinated drinking water, industrial agriculture, pesticides, sanitation, and antibiotics, while improving our lives in many ways, have created unforeseen health challenges. Alcohol, stress, and the high-fat/high-sugar Western diet compound the problem by suppressing what essential gut flora we do have, leading to a hyperreactive immune system primed for autoimmune disease and allergies.

If you suffer from any of the conditions mentioned in this chapter, the Live Dirty, Eat Clean Plan will give you step-by-step guidance on how to re-create some of the microbial exposure you might have missed out on as a child, and reveal which lifestyle choices enhance rather than suppress gut flora.

A Change of Scenery Outside . . . and Inside

Since our internal microbial landscape is in large part determined by our external environment, it's not surprising that relocating from a less antiseptic habitat to a super-clean one, or vice versa, can alter your microbiome and trigger disease. People from less developed countries have a heightened risk for developing Crohn's and other autoimmune illnesses when they move to the United States, especially when they move at a young age.

I diagnosed Anjali with Crohn's disease two years after she moved to the United States from India to attend college. She grew up in a strict vegetarian household where her mother or one of her aunts cooked plant-based meals from scratch with plenty of anti-inflammatory spices like turmeric, that were shared by multiple generations of her extended family living together in the same household. When she moved to the United States, she continued to eat a vegetarian diet, but pretty much lived on pizza and the contents of the vending machines at school. She developed adult acne, acid reflux, and indigestion that eventually turned into bloody diarrhea and severe ulceration throughout most of her colon and small intestine.

Anjali had never heard of Crohn's disease and didn't know anyone who had it, but her case was one of the most severe I had ever seen. We eventually got her into remission using a combination of conventional medication and drastic dietary modification, but she still feels best when she spends the summers in India eating her mother's cooking.

Atsenash grew up in Ethiopia, raised by her grandparents after her father died and her mother immigrated to the United States. At thirteen, she moved to the Midwest and was reunited with her mother, adopting a thoroughly American diet in an attempt to fit in with her teenage peers. Burgers and fries were the norm, but they were completely foreign to her, having grown up on a traditional Ethiopian diet that included the cereal grain teff, chili-spiced lentils, and greens. Her gastrointestinal (GI) tract quickly revolted, and by the time I met her ten years into her diagnosis of ulcerative colitis, her colon had been removed because of severe colitis unresponsive to even the most potent medical therapy.

It would seem that the protective effect of growing up in a rural environment with lots of microbes is no match for the detrimental effects of the Western diet and a super-sanitized lifestyle. But migration or travel in the other direction has its drawbacks, too. Many of my patients develop serious GI issues after overseas assignments with the Peace Corps or State Department. The symptoms usually develop after a bout of dysentery, which never quite resolves, and months later, investigation typically reveals chronic inflammation in the gut.

Another common scenario is traveler's diarrhea that overstays its welcome after a spring break trip to Mexico or the Caribbean, eventually morphing into Crohn's, ulcerative colitis, or post-infectious irritable bowel syndrome over the ensuing months or years (more on how and why that happens in Chapter 5 on dysbiosis).

Kerry was a healthy twenty-two-year-old who joined the Peace Corps after graduating from college and was assigned to a rural part of Ghana. She lived, worked, and ate with a family in the village, but unlike her host family, who were well acclimatized to the local microscopic flora and fauna, Kerry suffered multiple severe episodes of diarrhea, abdominal pain, nausea, and vomiting in the two years she was there. She was ultimately diagnosed with giardia as well as amebiasis—two well-known GI pathogens.

When she returned to the United States, the acute episodes resolved, but Kerry's bowel movements never returned to normal. She continued to have multiple soft stools daily, accompanied by abdominal cramping, and she started seeing blood in her stool a few times a week. Six months after returning home she came to see me about her symptoms. Stool studies at a reputable parasitology lab didn't reveal any active infection, so I recommended we take a closer look at her digestive tract. On colonoscopy she had confluent ulceration throughout the bottom half of her colon, consistent with a diagnosis of ulcerative colitis, which was also confirmed by biopsies. Kerry had no family history of ulcerative colitis or other autoimmune diseases, and no risk factors for developing IBD other than her GI distress while in Ghana. Her Western microbiome was simply unable to handle the onslaught of changes induced by the two parasites and the result was chronic inflammation.

Timing is everything when it comes to microbial exposure. Coming in contact with lots of germs when you're quite young can be a good thing, but when it happens suddenly as an adult . . . not so much. That's when invading pathogens can disrupt our delicate bacterial balance, crowding out essential species that are never completely restored.

So, Where Do Our Genes Come In?

Many diseases that run in families that we thought were primarily genetic, such as heart disease and some forms of cancer, turn out to be hugely influenced by gut bacteria. It's the complex and poorly understood interaction among your genes, your environment, and your immune system that ultimately determines whether you end up sick or not.

Epigenetics is the study of how our environment affects heritable traits without changing the actual DNA material in our genes. It's the classic nature-versus-nurture question: how much of who we are is a result of the genes we inherit, versus the environment we live in?

In fact, which gut bacteria you end up with may be even more im-

WHAT WE'RE FINDING is that the environment living inside us—our microbiome—has one of the biggest impacts on our genes, turning them on and off and determining which ones are ultimately expressed as disease.

portant than which genes you inherit. This is an empowering way of looking at disease, since we can't change our real family, but we *can* change our microbial family.

The vast majority of people with IBD don't have a family history of the disease or any identifiable genetic susceptibility, but that's not true for everyone. People of Eastern European Ashkenazi Jewish descent have a four- to fivefold increased risk of developing Crohn's, which is explained in part by a genetic variant that causes their immune system to overreact to gut flora. There are more than one hundred gene mutations associated with Crohn's, but gene abnormalities alone aren't enough to cause disease. It's triggers in the environment that ultimately unmask the genetic risk and lead to symptoms. We're getting better at identifying those triggers and are realizing that most of them involve changes in gut bacteria. In fact, we can produce Crohn's in mice by transferring gut bacteria from affected mice to healthy, germ-free mice, confirming that the microbiome plays an important, if not causative, role.

Too Clean on the Inside?

There's such a strong link between antibiotic use and digestive issues that it's literally the first question I ask new patients in my practice. In *Gutbliss* I wrote about the correlation between regular use of antibiotics and the development of bloating, yeast infections, and other types of microbial discord known as dysbiosis, and in this book I've devoted a whole chapter to it (see Chapter 5). But the idea that antibiotics might cause serious autoimmune illnesses like Crohn's and ulcerative colitis is a relatively new concept. It's also a troubling one, because our threshold for prescribing antibiotics is dangerously low. What's more, for decades we've been using antibiotics to treat flare-ups of these diseases! Could the very drugs we've so readily dispensed be part of the reason we're seeing such a dramatic increase in these modern plagues?

Being treated with antibiotics in your first year of life is associated with a threefold increase in risk for IBD compared to children who haven't received antibiotics, and the risk seems to increase the more antibiotics you receive. In countries like Canada and Finland where antibiotics are widely available, the incidence of IBD in children has steadily increased about 5 percent to 8 percent annually. Studies from the United States, including a meta-analysis of more than seven thousand patients by researchers at Mount Sinai Hospital, confirm that the risk of IBD from antibiotics is highest in children, but also show an increase in new-onset Crohn's in adults who've taken antibiotics in the months before diagnosis. All antibiotics except penicillin have been implicated, but, ironically, the ones most commonly used to treat Crohn's—metronidazole and fluoroquinolones like Ciprofloxacin—confer the highest risk.

Extensive antibiotic use wipes out large amounts of bacteria, including both protective and pathogenic species. As luck would have it, the bad bacteria are often hardier than the good ones and more likely to survive the antibiotic assault. They end up multiplying and filling the gap created by the overall loss in numbers, which creates the typical profile seen in people with IBD: an overall decrease in diversity of gut bacteria, higher levels of pathogenic species, and lower levels of protective ones.

Novel Ways to Rewild Yourself

In patients with illnesses like Crohn's, attempts to dampen the immune system without the risk of infection that characterizes most immune-suppressing drugs has led to a novel type of therapy: inoculation with parasites. The theory is that controlled infection with helminths such as hookworms can restore the body's autoimmune system to a more balanced state, decreasing the response to stimuli and reducing inflammation in the gut. While hookworm therapy isn't without risk (including rashes, itching, anemia, diarrhea, and overwhelming infection), some studies have shown an overall benefit for conditions such as Crohn's, MS, asthma, and certain types of allergies. The worms are introduced as eggs that the patient drinks in a salty solution, and the inoculum is kept to a low level so as to avoid severe infection, which can actually trigger inflammation.

Some researchers are now using pig whipworms instead of hookworms, which are unable to reproduce in humans and therefore need to be ingested every few weeks, but don't have the risk of overwhelming chronic infection. In one trial involving fifty-four patients with ulcerative colitis, 43 percent of those who received pig whipworm eggs improved, compared to only 17 percent of those who didn't. In a second trial involving Crohn's disease patients, whipworm eggs were administered every three weeks. After six months of therapy, almost 80 percent of the patients had significantly reduced disease activity, and 72 percent had gone into a complete remission.

Helminthic therapy is still in the experimental stages, but under the right circumstances it may ultimately prove to be a step in the right direction toward rewilding ourselves and reclaiming our health.

Clean Food as Medicine

The most surprising thing about chronic inflammatory digestive disorders such as Crohn's and ulcerative colitis may be the fact that the medical community still has a hard time accepting the idea that what we put into our digestive tract has any influence at all on what goes on inside it or what comes out the other end.

I have to confess that years ago when I was practicing at a teaching hospital and seeing patients with stubborn cases of IBD, I thought that way, too. I wholeheartedly believed in the superiority and necessity of pharmaceutical intervention. Patients who insisted on treating their disease naturally using diet and supplements made me nervous. I was constantly expecting their condition to worsen and their disease to flare. Sometimes that happened. But in many cases it didn't. And over time, with the help of many wonderful patients who allowed me to fiddle with their food, it became clear that healing inflammation in the gut by altering the microbiome through diet was a realistic and worthwhile goal.

Annette is a patient born in Argentina whom I saw in consultation for Crohn's disease. Like most people from that part of the world, she received the bacillus Calmette–Guérin, or BCG, vaccine against tuberculosis as a child. Since the vaccine is prepared from a strain of live tuberculosis that has lost its virulence in humans, one of the possible side effects is a false positive skin test for tuberculosis, which is exactly what happened to Annette when she was screened for tuberculosis in middle school. As a result of the positive test, she was treated for active tuberculosis infection with three antibiotics for a total of nine months, even though she never had any signs or symptoms of tuberculosis, and an X-ray of her lungs failed to show any evidence of the disease.

In her senior year of high school Annette developed abdominal pain, diarrhea, and weight loss. She was diagnosed with Crohn's disease and started on a series of drugs that included immune-modulating agents. Her disease improved significantly, although she continued to have occasional episodes of mild abdominal pain and difficulty gaining weight. Ten years after being diagnosed with Crohn's, Annette decided she wanted to start a family. She and her husband weren't comfortable with her getting pregnant on the medications she was taking because of the potential risk to the fetus, so before trying to conceive she embarked on a dietary regimen that excluded processed foods, most grains, and refined sugar that had worked for a friend with IBD. The diet worked for Annette, too, and within four months she had successfully tapered off all her medications.

Her former gastroenterologist had recommended she resume all her medications immediately after her pregnancy, but she was still in remission and feeling well a year after delivering a healthy baby boy, and she wanted to continue trying to control her Crohn's with diet alone. I liberalized her diet a bit, adding in some of the things she missed and wanted to try to reintroduce, and three years after starting the diet Annette remains in remission on no medications.

I still have a prescription pad, but I try to use it as little as possible—not because the drugs don't work but because risks like infection and cancer and the fact that many of these drugs cross the placenta and are present in breast milk tend to outweigh the benefits for the more effective therapies. The less potent drugs have fewer side effects, but they also don't work as well—in fact, some have a response rate that's the same as treatment with a placebo, or sugar pill! Interestingly, we use the same pool of drugs to treat IBD that we employ for other autoimmune conditions such as rheumatoid arthritis and psoriasis, and the dietary therapy that works so well for our patients' intestinal problems frequently improves their other coexisting autoimmune problems, suggesting a common mechanism of causation and cure.

Most of my patients are interested in a more holistic approach and believe, as I do, in the concept of food as medicine. Our usual practice is to start with dietary modification, along with robust probiotics (live beneficial bacteria that you'll learn more about in Chapter 12), adding in medications with low toxicity if needed and occasionally graduating to the bigger-gun drugs if the dietary changes and more benign therapies aren't helping. We also incorporate biofeedback to teach patients how to relieve spasm in the involuntary muscles of their digestive tracts through mind-body techniques of guided meditation and visualization. So it really is a pyramid approach, with nutritional therapy and rehabilitation of the microbiome being the foundation on which everything else rests.

For most people, there really is no downside to using food as medicine, and there are clearly countless other benefits to eating a healthy diet besides putting your IBD into remission. But I do occasionally have patients whose disease is so severe that I recommend cooling things down with stronger conventional therapy first before embarking on the slower pace of dietary change. Some patients are just too sick and need faster-acting and more potent drugs. Even then, my goal is always to transition off those drugs as quickly as possible once the inflammation has improved, and to try to maintain the results with diet and lifestyle whenever possible.

A few years ago we embarked on a nutritional study in our practice to assess the effectiveness of a low-complex-carbohydrate diet in improving the quality of life and reducing the frequency and severity of flare-ups in patients with IBD. The diet excluded most grains, sugars, and starches but included healthy carbohydrates such as fruits, vegetables, and legumes. It is the basis for what I recommend in the Live Dirty, Eat Clean Plan. We analyzed data from twelve patients who had followed the diet for a minimum of sixty days, looking at quality of life and disease activity before and after the diet, including healing of gut inflammation. Three of the patients had ulcerative colitis and nine had Crohn's disease, with an average of ten years since diagnosis. About half of the patients had disease severe enough to have required previous surgery.

All twelve patients reported that the diet helped their symptoms, and ten out of twelve described a dramatic improvement. Two-thirds (eight out of twelve) were able to stop or decrease their medications after adopting the diet. Eight patients underwent colonoscopy during the study period, and six of them showed significant healing of their inflammation, with no additional intervention other than the dietary changes. The average time to see improvement after starting the diet was thirty-eight days, although there was a wide range: some patients reported significant improvement after as little as three days, while it took some patients four months to notice a difference in their symptoms.

Our study was small, but our results confirmed what I knew to be true from clinical observation: dietary modification works and is a viable option for the treatment of IBD, either as primary therapy or in combination with medication. Not only can it improve symptoms and allow a reduction or discontinuation of drugs, but it can also lead to actual healing of the inflammation in the gut. Our strong hunch is that these changes are mediated through alterations in gut bacteria.

Bottom line: one of the most powerful tools in preventing and treating our modern plagues might be the food we eat, since that's what determines which bacteria grow in our gut garden. In my Live Dirty, Eat Clean Plan, I'll give you a step-by-step road map for implementing these changes in your own life, balancing your microbiome, and creating long-lasting good health along the way.

Reclaiming Our Health by Rethinking "Clean"

When most people think about germs, they think of disease and poverty in faraway places, or of families and their livestock living ten to a hut, with limited access to clean water and medical care and the next pandemic just one unwashed hand away. While it's true that infectious diseases like cholera and tuberculosis still plague poorer countries, in the more developed world it's actually the lack of germs that's making many of us sick. As the next chapter will show, some of our "medical miracles," when used indiscriminately, can end up contributing to, rather than curing, disease.

CHAPTER 4

||||||||||||||||||||||||||||||||||||||||||||

Pharmageddon and the Antibiotic Paradox

THERE'S NO QUESTION that Alexander Fleming's discovery of penicillin in 1928 is still one of the greatest contributions to medicine. It could have prevented events like the Great Plague of the 1600s, which wiped out a quarter of the population of Europe. Antibiotics prevent death from serious infection every day, sparing the human race untold misery. But in our current climate of overdiagnosis and overtreatment, they're also used indiscriminately for a wide variety of minor, self-limited conditions. Conservative estimates suggest that almost half of all antibiotic use is inappropriate, resulting in increased side effects, higher costs, and resistance to antibiotics that threatens to plunge us back into the dark ages of medicine, before we had these drugs at our disposal.

Survival of the Fittest

Antibiotics kill bacteria by penetrating their protective outer membrane and gaining access to their insides. But repeated use can actually make bacteria stronger, the same way training with super-fast teammates can make you a better runner. Genetic mutations allow some bacteria to grow thicker membranes that prevent access, while others adapt by producing toxins that neutralize antibiotics or borrow drug-resistant genes from neighboring bacteria that allow them to survive even the deadliest attacks.

With all these guerrilla tactics at our microbes' disposal, it's not surprising that what we thought was an endless pipeline of new miracle antibiotics is now running dry. Resistant superbugs kill thousands of people every year and cause illness in two million more in the United States alone. Hard-to-treat infections acquired in the hospital—the training ground for resistant superbugs—kill more Americans every year than murders and car accidents combined.

Yet we keep sidestepping the pressing issue of more judicious antibiotic use, believing we can still use these drugs indiscriminately and somehow also manage to stay ahead of our microbial hackers, outsmarting them by creating drugs that will stop them in their tracks and remain effective. It hasn't happened yet and it probably never will, because microbes are in the business of survival, which means adapting to whatever inhospitable environment they find themselves in and figuring out how to evade it.

What You Don't Know Can Hurt You

The truth is, until recently we had no idea that there were real risks to systematically killing off gut bacteria. Most of us doing the prescribing did so based on the prevailing—but grossly inaccurate—premise that antibiotics are good and germs are bad; therefore, killing off bacteria should lead to better health.

Most of the antibiotics we use today have activity against a broad spectrum of bacteria. That's desirable in our current medical climate of "shoot first, ask questions later" and would make sense if the risks of antibiotics didn't outweigh their benefits. But we now know that's hardly the case. Side effects like nausea, vomiting, diarrhea, skin rashes, and stomachaches pale in comparison to the main risks of antibiotics: indiscriminate elimination of droves of your essential bacteria, and the hard-to-treat illnesses that ensue as a result. We'll be exploring those illnesses in detail in the next chapter.

Let's take a look at one of the most deadly and increasingly prevalent consequences of antibiotic use that's now a major public health crisis.

Germs Gone Wild

Clostridium difficile, also known as *C. diff*, is a bacterium that can wreak serious havoc in the GI tract. It's the cause of one-third of all cases of antibiotic-associated diarrhea (AAD) and of most cases of pseudomembranous colitis, a severe and sometimes deadly form of AAD. *C. diff* is endemic in hospitals, where health care workers unwittingly transmit it from patient to patient, leading to colonization rates of up to 50 percent in hospitals and 10 percent in chronic care facilities. About 2 percent of healthy asymptomatic people in the community also harbor *C. diff*, and some of us are colonized with it at birth.

The first step in acquiring *C. diff* infection is alteration of your normal gut flora through administration of antibiotics. Clindamycin was the first antibiotic associated with *C. diff*, but virtually any antibiotic can cause it, and so can many chemotherapy agents. The changes in your microbiome after treatment with these drugs leave you vulnerable to bacteria like *C. diff* multiplying.

The second step is acquisition, which can occur through contact with a hospitalized patient, health care worker, or asymptomatic carrier. *C. diff* bacteria and their spores are found in feces and can infect people who touch contaminated surfaces and then touch their mouth. Health care workers who don't wash their hands carefully can spread the bacteria, creating a mini pandemic among patients they've been in contact with. In addition to the high rates in hospitalized patients, we're seeing more and more community-acquired *C. diff*, suggesting that colonization rates outside the hospital setting are rising.

After acquisition, the third step is either development of disease or asymptomatic colonization. Your age, general level of health, and immune status all play a role in determining whether or not you end up sick. Long-term use of acid-suppressing drugs is a major risk factor for developing *C. diff*, since stomach acid is one of the body's main defenses against invading bacteria. People taking these drugs are more likely to have recurrent infection and poorer outcomes, including a higher risk of dying from *C. diff*, compared to people not on acid suppression.

In those who become infected, *C. diff* proliferates in the gut, releasing toxins that cause severe diarrhea, cramping, and bloating, and in some cases more serious illnesses like pseudomembranous colitis. Because of widespread use of antibiotics, *C. diff* infection now affects 1 percent of all hospitalized patients in the United States, with a total of 250,000 infections per year and fourteen thousand deaths. Ironically, our main approach to *C. diff* infection has been to treat it with more antibiotics—and not surprisingly, we're seeing a tremendous increase in the number of infections that are refractory, or resistant, to standard treatment.

Resistant *C. diff* has led to a novel type of therapy: fecal transplants that involve transferring stool from healthy donors into the digestive tract of the person infected with *C. diff*. A study published in the *New England Journal of Medicine* showed that fecal transplants were far more effective in clearing up recurrent *C. diff* infection than standard antibiotic therapy, reinforcing the idea of bugs over drugs for good digestive health. In Chapter 13, I'll tell you everything you ever wanted to know about fecal transplants but were afraid to ask, including the risks and benefits, and how to perform one in the privacy of your own home.

Rising rates of community-acquired *C. diff* infection have definitely increased awareness about the dangers of unnecessary antibiotic use, but the number of people receiving these drugs inappropriately is still quite shocking, as are the consequences we'll be discussing in the next chapter.

Fat Farming

We've been using antibiotics to fatten up farm animals for more than half a century, since we figured out that adding antibiotics to livestock feed makes the animals gain weight faster. The same thing may be happening to those of us who eat those antibiotic-fed animals. Antibiotics can selectively enhance the growth of microbes that are able to extract more energy from food. Studies have shown that giving low-dose antibiotics to baby mice for just a few weeks can make them obese in later life (not to mention contribute to disease), and the rise in obesity and modern plagues in the United States closely parallels the practice of widespread antibiotic use in factory farming. We'll talk more about this controversial method of growth promotion and its implications for our health in Chapter 7, "Modern Microbial Disruptors."

Antibiotic Overkill

Between 2000 and 2010, global antibiotic use increased by 35 percent. Although India uses the most antibiotics worldwide, the United States ranks number one in per capita consumption, with a whopping one hundred million prescriptions written every year during adult outpatient visits alone. The average American child will receive about seventeen courses of antibiotics by his or her eighteenth birthday, mostly for illnesses that don't require any treatment. Ear infections are a great example of antibiotic overkill. Most are viral but are treated with antibiotics "just in case" there is a bacterial component—a strategy that does nothing to speed recovery and can lead to side effects like diarrhea and stomachaches that actually make children feel worse. A Harvard study on the treatment of sore throats in more than four thousand children found that the rate of treatment with antibiotics greatly exceeded the rate of positive results, and that testing for *Strep* and other pathogens was done less than half the time in children who were prescribed antibiotics.

There are some infections that definitely require antibiotic treatment, but more often the need for antibiotics is a gray area. A study published in the journal *Pediatrics* found that pediatricians prescribed antibiotics 62 percent of the time when they perceived that parents expected them to be prescribed, and only 7 percent of the time when they thought parents didn't, suggesting that the need for antibiotics is almost always optional.

It's not just children who are being overtreated. Two out of every three adults who see a health practitioner for cold or flu symptoms are prescribed antibiotics, which 80 percent of the time don't meet Centers for Disease Control and Prevention (CDC) guidelines for antibiotic therapy. When I ask my patients about previous antibiotic use, they usually respond that they took "a normal amount," but after I have them add up every prescription, they're often shocked to realize just how much "normal" really is.

In my Live Dirty, Eat Clean Plan, I'll give you clear strategies for avoiding the pitfall of unnecessary antibiotics, including the ten most important questions to ask your doctor if you've been prescribed an antibiotic.

An Ounce of Prevention Isn't Always Worth a Pound of Cure

Treating people who have symptoms, regardless of whether they really need an antibiotic, is a bad idea. But using antibiotics to suppress bacteria in asymptomatic people on the off chance that they *may* get sick in the future is an even worse one. Unfortunately, such prophylactic or preventive use is now common practice for all sorts of situations, including urinary tract symptoms, indwelling catheters, elective surgery, childbirth, and some dental procedures. In addition, long-term use of antibiotics to dampen the immune system as an optimistic but unproven way of improving symptoms has become standard of care for chronic inflammatory conditions like asthma, acne, arthritis, and Crohn's disease. Our default seems to have become: when in doubt, treat with an antibiotic.

For most elective procedures, the risk of an antibiotic-associated complication such as severe diarrhea, a rash, or even potentially deadly *C. diff* outweighs the risk of infection. Many of the guidelines that recommend prophylactic antibiotics for invasive procedures were written years ago, before we knew the real risks of antibiotics, and they haven't been recently revised or revisited. If you've been told to take an antibiotic prior to a procedure, be sure to read Chapter 11, "A Rewilding Approach to Illness," before agreeing, and ask whether a reasonable option instead could be careful observation and rapid intervention if you were to get an infection.

Prescribing antibiotics prophylactically can actually make us sicker—lengthening our recovery time and putting us at increased risk for more serious infection by killing off essential protective bacteria along with any pathogens, leaving us less prepared for the next infection.

When Less Is More

Carol came to see me complaining of bloating and unpredictable bouts of diarrhea. She'd been on so many courses of antibiotics for recurrent sinus infections that her doctor had started putting her on "suppressive" antibiotic treatment every fall in the misguided hope of staving off yet another sinus infection. Although she was still getting six or seven severe infections a year, he reasoned that it would probably have been worse without the prophylactic antibiotics. He also told her that she likely had something wrong with her immune system, and that was why she was sick so often. However, a thorough evaluation with an immunologist revealed no immune system abnormalities other than one weakened by overexposure to antimicrobial drugs.

I told Carol that it was completely abnormal and unacceptable for her to have so many sinus infections, and that I wouldn't be able to do anything for her bloating and diarrhea until we addressed the antibiotic use, which was almost certainly the cause of both her bowel and sinus problems. She was incredulous at the suggestion that the very drugs she'd grown to depend on could actually be contributing to, rather than curing, her sinusitis. It took a long time to convince Carol to stop taking antibiotics and the nasal steroid sprays she used daily that were suppressing the healthy flora of her sinus passages. Every few months she would call and preface the conversation with, "Don't be mad, but I had to take another round of antibiotics" as she related yet another horrible sinus infection that necessitated treatment.

Carol's immunologist and I finally persuaded her to try another approach, and after suffering through several infections with just antihistamines, we started to see light at the end of the tunnel. I don't see Carol anymore because when she stopped taking the antibiotics, her GI symptoms eventually resolved along with her chronic sinusitis!

Carol's experience is all too common and illustrates how frequent antibiotic use can set you on a path of habitual infection. Chronic sinusitis sufferers have an average of nine hundred bacterial strains in their nasal passages, whereas those who are not have closer to twelve hundred strains. The presence of the additional strains is what's actually protecting the healthy people. Frequent antibiotic use in people with chronic sinusitis wipes out those essential protective strains, making them more, not less, susceptible to recurrent infection and perpetuating the cycle of . . . you guessed it . . . more antibiotics. It can be hard to say no to something you've been told is therapeutic, but if you're not getting better, it's important to ask yourself why, and to consider whether "the cure" might actually be part of the cause.

Breaking the Cycle

When Melody came to my office, she had been experiencing symptoms consistent with a urinary tract infection, including burning and frequent urination, every couple of months for the last several years. Each time this happened, she would call her physician's office, and the very nice receptionist would call in a prescription for an antibiotic for her. No urinalysis or culture was ordered to determine whether she had an infection and, if so, what kind of bacteria was causing it, nor was she examined to see if she had a fever, or just to get a sense of how sick she really was.

Melody had a long history of interstitial cystitis, a chronic inflammatory condition of the bladder associated with urgency and frequency, and the only tool she had ever been given to manage her chronic bladder symptoms was antibiotics. Now she was paying the price. Her bladder, an area that's usually pretty sterile, had become colonized with antibiotic-resistant strains of bacteria as a result of all her antibiotic use. Each dose of antibiotics brought her temporary relief but ultimately compounded the problem, driving her bacteria to become more and more resistant.

Melody's was a relatively easy fix: a major dietary rehab to get rid of all the sugar and bread she was eating that was also feeding the wrong types of bacteria in her bladder, and D-mannose, a naturally occurring carbohydrate, that relieved her urinary symptoms. I'll take you step-by-step through what to do for your own urinary tract symptoms and other common infections in Chapter 11, "A Rewilding Approach to Illness."

Not everyone is as receptive to discontinuing antibiotics or willing to embrace the dietary changes as wholeheartedly as Melody was, but most of my patients who commit to improving their microbiome do eventually see results. When people with dysbiosis consult me for treatment, one of the first things I ask them to do is agree not to take antibiotics unless absolutely necessary. You may be miserable for several weeks, but committing to breaking the cycle of recurrent antibiotic use is the most important step in restoring your microbiome and getting rid of your symptoms for good. High levels of essential bacteria, not antibiotics, are our best defense against the threat of infection.

If Carol's or Melody's story sounds familiar, the hardest part might be letting go of your antibiotic security blanket. Because it provides temporary, short-lived relief, you might still be clinging to the idea that it's part of the solution. I can understand that perspective, considering how these drugs have been marketed.

We've become so accustomed to reaching for an antibiotic when we're sick that it's a revelation for many of my patients to hear that it's possible to soldier through non-life-threatening infections without any antimicrobial therapy. The belief that there's always a quick-fix, low-risk option is what got us into this pickle in the first place, and clearly the way out is to adopt a different paradigm for dealing with being unwell. We have to radically change our expectations about illness and suffering, and indeed about health itself, accepting that a certain degree of inconvenience and periodic discomfort are part of normal life—and also part of strengthening our immune system.

Probiotics: Not a Cure-All, Either

Probiotics are live microorganisms that provide health benefits when consumed, but we're still in the early days of development for these products, and there aren't a lot of rigorous scientific studies or guidelines to tell us which ones are best for which specific diagnosis, how long we need to take them, and how much of them we should be taking. In Chapter 12, I'll provide an extensive guide to what we do know, and guidelines to help you decide if a probiotic might be helpful for you in restoring microbial balance.

Part of the challenge is that we're only able to culture and grow a small percentage of gut bacteria outside of the digestive tract, and fewer still can survive long enough in pill or powder form to prove truly beneficial. So although probiotics can be helpful in restoring microbial balance, they're not a panacea. It's inaccurate to tout them as a miracle antidote to antibiotics, which are a powerful force to be reckoned with in terms of their effects on the microbiome. A five-day course of a single broad-spectrum antimicrobial agent such as Ciprofloxacin can suppress up to a third of your gut bacteria. Because the microbiome is dynamic, many of those species will return to baseline levels, but more often than not, whole populations of gut bacteria remain low long after treatment has ended, despite months of probiotic therapy. That's why I try to stress to my patients the importance of antibiotic avoidance and a healthy diet instead of just relying on microbial replacement via probiotics. Destroying your gut bacteria and then trying to replenish them with a probiotic is like draining a full bathtub and replacing the contents with a single cup of water—it's literally a drop in the bucket.

The reality is that most of us with a healthy, balanced microbiome can weather the storm of an antibiotic every few years, but we may have a difficult time recovering from persistent excessive use. The drugs are just too potent. And for those of us who've fed our microbes a steady diet of processed food, our ability to bounce back from antibiotics is even more limited. So, avoidance of antibiotics is absolutely the number one strategy for keeping your microbiome healthy. I'll discuss other common prescription and over-the-counter medications that threaten microbial health in Chapter 11, "A Rewilding Approach to Illness."

Pharmageddon

Pharmageddon is psychiatrist David Healy, MD's searing indictment of the overuse of prescription medication. It's a forceful argument against the pharmaceuticalization of health care, and links this dangerous trend to an increase in deaths and disabilities. What he describes is a real-life dystopian society where the medical and pharmaceutical industries have an overall detrimental effect on human health, and scientific advances do more harm than good. Thankfully, Pharmageddon hasn't yet fully arrived, but if antibiotic-prescribing habits are any indication, it's rapidly approaching.

CHAPTER 5

|||||||||||||||||||||||||||||||||||||||||||

Dysbiosis—Do You Have It?

MOST OF THE PEOPLE who walk into my office today describe problems entirely different from those I saw twenty years ago when I finished my medical training. Back then, most of my patients were suffering from conditions such as acid reflux, bleeding ulcers, gallstones, diverticulitis, colitis, and the occasional colon cancer. These were easily diagnosable diseases that you could see and touch; they were readily apparent on standard testing, with straightforward and generally effective treatment.

Over the last few years, I've been witness to an epidemic of hard-to-diagnose, vague, and seemingly unrelated manifestations in people who don't really have disease in the classic sense. What they have is symptoms. Almost all of them have seen at least one doctor (and most have been to several), and many have been told that their symptoms are being caused by stress or by their imagination.

Fortunately, our body has its own innate sense of when something is wrong, and it usually encourages us to seek answers and solutions, even when mainstream medicine is telling us we're fine or is failing us in other ways. It's one of the reasons I wrote this book—to empower my fellow citizen scientists and remind them that, ultimately, our bodies have a wisdom that should not be ignored.

Murky Symptoms and a Common Thread

For a long time, I puzzled over what I was hearing from my patients. They complained of bloating, abdominal pain, smelly gas, rashes, rosacea, food intolerances, "weird-looking" stools, fatigue, brain fog, frequent infections, and generally just feeling "off." Some had been given the unsatisfying label of irritable bowel syndrome (IBS), a diagnosis that confirms you have gastrointestinal (GI) symptoms and don't feel well but doesn't attempt to explain why.

I took their complaints seriously and performed thorough investigations of their digestive tracts, looking for clues and answers. I examined their stomachs with my endoscope, got up close and personal with their colons with my colonoscope, and took pictures of their small intestine (where not much happens, but I wanted to take a look just in case) with an ingestible video capsule. I ordered gallbladder tests and CAT (computerized axial tomography) scans and lots of blood work. Invariably it would all come back normal. Yet it was clear that something was terribly wrong. My patients weren't crazy or hypochondriacs. Their symptoms just didn't fit the typical profile of digestive disease we were used to seeing, and the traditional tools we had for diagnosing and treating them weren't getting the job done.

Despite the wide range of symptoms patients reported, one shared experience kept popping up again and again. At first I thought it was coincidence, but as I got into the habit of asking about past medications (which sometimes necessitated tracking down elderly parents to get details of their grown children's childhood ailments and treatment), and as our collective understanding of the importance of gut bacteria grew, a clear picture began to emerge. These patients had all, at some point in their lives, been prescribed a lot of antibiotics.

A New Type of Disease

These patients' heavy antibiotic use had culminated in serious imbalance in their gut bacteria—a condition called dysbiosis. Dysbiosis is an alteration of the microbial community that diminishes a person's essential population of good bacteria and allows pathogenic (bad) bacteria that are normally present in low amounts to flourish—in essence, it is a *microbial imbalance in or on your body.* It can be a challenging diagnosis to make. There are a few tests that may provide supporting evidence, but dysbiosis is primarily a clinical diagnosis based on careful history taking and familiarity with the spectrum of disorders that can result from damage to the microbiome.

Because you can't see it or touch it the way you can most digestive diseases, and because it's largely a result of our own overzealous medical practices, mainstream medicine is only now beginning to recognize dysbiosis as a real condition, despite the fact that millions of people suffer from it. Getting a vaginal yeast infection or thrush in your mouth after a round of antibiotics is a classic example of localized dysbiosis: your native yeast population proliferates unchecked after the antibiotic destroys large numbers of essential bacteria. Severe dysbiosis may manifest as more serious disease that can affect the entire body, like the autoimmune diseases we discussed in Chapter 3.

These days, dysbiosis is the most common disorder I see in my gastroenterology practice. It's a virtual epidemic of patients who wish they could turn back time and undo the years of antibiotics they took for acne, sinus infections, or whatever other non-life-threatening condition they were treated for, without any awareness of the long-term risks.

Dysbiosis affects up to thirty million Americans, in large part because the factors that damage our gut bacteria are so ubiquitous. Antibiotics aren't the only threat to our microbiome. Our food and drink, daily meds, and stressful, overscheduled lives can all be major microbial disruptors. Dysbiosis is often the root cause behind many poorly under-

TABLE 5–1 • Causes of Dysbiosis

- Antibiotics
- PPIs (proton pump inhibitors)/antacids
- NSAIDs (nonsteroidal anti-inflammatory drugs)
- BCP (birth control pills)/hormones
- Steroids
- Chemotherapy
- Artificial sweeteners
- Too much sugar and fat
- Not enough fiber
- Alcohol
- Stress
- Infections

stood and increasingly common medical conditions like leaky gut, irritable bowel syndrome, and several autoimmune disorders, and it also provides a compelling explanation for why some people have such a hard time losing weight—a topic we'll explore in detail in the next chapter. If you've suffered from a variety of symptoms that have been difficult to diagnose, or have multiple ailments and wondered about a common cause, dysbiosis may be the explanation you've been looking for.

Detecting Dysbiosis:
Is Your Medicine Cabinet a Menace?

You may think of your medicine cabinet as the place to go for solutions to what ails you, but when it comes to dysbiosis, it's often the source of the problem. We've talked above and in the previous chapter about the devastating consequences of too many antibiotics, but lots of other drugs, both over-the-counter and prescription, can wreak havoc on your microbiome by killing off irreplaceable amounts of bacteria, changing the pH of the gut in a way that favors overgrowth of the wrong species, or damaging the gut lining and allowing bacteria access to areas where they normally shouldn't be.

Are You Missing Stomach Acid?

Over-the-counter antacids, H2 receptor antagonists, and proton pump inhibitors (PPIs) all work single-mindedly toward the same goal: blocking your stomach acid. That might bring relief if you have acid reflux, but it comes at a price. Stomach acid is one of our main defenses against undesirable bacteria that enter the body through the mouth. Acid-blocking drugs transform the normally inhospitable acidic environment of the stomach into a friendly place for bacteria to grow and multiply, potentially throwing off your microbial balance and causing dysbiosis.

Acid-blocking drugs can also lead to overgrowth of undesirable bacteria in the small intestine, causing symptoms of gas, bloating, and belching that can mimic the signs of acid reflux in someone who's already being treated—a classic example of how pharmaceutical intervention for one problem can actually create disease elsewhere. Lifestyle modifications—such as cutting down on caffeine, dairy, and alcohol and eating more plants and less fat—will help banish your reflux and boost your microbes without swapping one problem for another.

Acid suppressive therapy also puts you at increased risk for pneumonia and dreaded *Clostridium difficile* that would normally be repelled by stomach acid, and it increases your overall risk for infection by changing the bacterial makeup of the gut. Taking an antibiotic when you're on a PPI adds insult to injury in terms of damage to your microbiome and significantly increases your risk for developing dysbiosis.

In infants, the valve between the esophagus and stomach sometimes isn't fully functional at birth, which can lead to acid refluxing up from the stomach into the esophagus, causing heartburn and spit-up after eating. The simple solution is to give your baby small frequent feedings and keep your little one upright for at least an hour after. But so many parents are simply handed a prescription for some type of acid suppression instead—a particularly egregious practice in babies, whose precious microbes are just blossoming. Those kids often end up with more than their share of upper respiratory tract infections, which leads to antibiotics on top of the acid suppression, setting them up for a lifetime of problems. Some parents—and physicians—aren't well informed about these complex interactions among medications, microbes, and our health. It's why you need to be absolutely vigilant about researching and questioning every recommended pharmaceutical intervention for you and your family, and not assume that the outcome will be better health.

Are NSAIDs Making Holes in Your Gut?

Nonsteroidal anti-inflammatory drugs (NSAIDs) don't have direct antimicrobial activity, but they can cause ulceration and increase the intestinal permeability of the lining of the gut, which allows bacteria to translocate through and damage the mucosa—a major contributor to the phenomenon of leaky gut. Increased intestinal permeability is a microscopic version of the gastric ulcers we see from these drugs. Unlike bleeding ulcers, leaky gut doesn't have a high mortality rate, but it can cause untold misery and suffering as a result of the symptoms that may ensue once the intestinal lining is damaged. We'll wade through the murky waters of leaky gut later in this chapter.

Are Hormones Wreaking Havoc?

Birth control pills are the most common form of contraception in the United States today and are used by millions of women for additional reasons besides preventing pregnancy, such as to decrease menstrual cramps, clear up acne, treat endometriosis, and reduce symptoms of premenstrual syndrome. Unfortunately, both birth control pills and hormone replacement therapy increase estrogen levels, which affect your microbial ecosystem and can lead to chronic yeast infections and other signs of dysbiosis. Giving up birth control pills can be tricky— it's a convenient and effective form of contraception—but if you think you may have dysbiosis, it may be time to look for a nonhormonal alternative.

Are You Over-suppressed by Steroids?

Corticosteroids such as prednisone are used to combat almost every form of inflammation, although because of their extensive side-effect profile and ability to dampen the immune system, they're also a major source of dysbiosis, disability, and even death. They're a danger to the microbiome because they suppress friendly bacteria and allow the pro-liferation of fungal species, which can be associated with severe forms of bacterial imbalance. A weakened immune system also makes steroid users more prone to infection.

Leslie came to see me for severe bloating, gas, and rectal itching. She had a normal abdominal exam but evidence of chronic fungal in-fection on her thumbs and several of her toenails and what looked like diaper rash under her arms and around her anus. She'd been on several short courses of high-dose steroids for asthma and had been using a hemorrhoid cream that contained steroids on the rash around her anus, which, not surprisingly, was getting worse. Her situation didn't require any microscopic evaluation. The manifestations of yeast overgrowth were written all over her body. Once we got rid of the offending steroid agents, her microbiome eventually bounced back and her bloating, gas, and rectal itching resolved.

Is Chemotherapy Killing Off Your Cells?

In an ideal world, chemotherapy would just kill cancer cells and leave the rest of your body alone. Unfortunately, however, when these powerful drugs do their work of poisoning cells, lots of microbial cells are affected, too. It may be why secondary cancers and autoimmune problems are so common after chemotherapy and why patients have such a hard time recovering and regaining their health after chemo treatment—the microbiome may take years to recover from this kind of toxic assault. If you're facing a serious cancer, you may not be able to avoid chemo, but paying careful attention to the health of your gut bacteria during and after chemo and feeding them the most nourishing food possible should be an integral part of your treatment plan.

Detecting Dysbiosis: Are You Being Poisoned by Your Food?

I have a very simple definition of food: something that nourishes you. That means it should nourish your gut bacteria, too, since a thriving microbiome is the key to good health.

In addition to needing specific essential raw materials and nutrients in order to survive, gut bacteria also need to be protected from toxins and chemicals in food, and from the wrong types of food, which can lead to the demise of essential bacteria and the proliferation of not so desirable species. My Live Dirty, Eat Clean Plan tells you exactly what to remove from your diet, and what to replace it with, to make sure you're feeding your microbes exactly what they need.

Are You Choosing Chemicals over Calories?

Artificial sweeteners claim to save you calories because they aren't absorbed by the small intestine, but they're still plenty sweet, and studies show that they may result in the release of just as much, if not more, insulin (the hormone that tells your cells to store extra calories as fat) as regular sugar. But weight gain isn't their only potential drawback; their effect on your microbiome is equally troubling. Artificial sweeteners are fermented by gut bacteria in the colon, which produces lots of bloat-causing gas, and a 2014 study published in the journal *Nature* suggests that they also damage gut bacteria in the process. So, if the story about artificial sweeteners seems too good to be true—sweetness without calories or side effects—it is.

Are You Feeding the Wrong Bacteria?

A sugary, starchy, fat-laden diet can send bad bacteria into a feeding frenzy and encourage growth of the wrong type of bacteria in your gut. Italian researchers compared children in Florence, Italy, eating a typical Western diet (high-fat/high-sugar) with a rural group in Burkina Faso eating fiber-rich legumes and vegetables. Gut bacteria were similar in the children when they were breast-fed babies, but as soon as they started to eat their local diet, significant differences emerged. The European group eating the high-fat/high-sugar diet had less microbial diversity and more species associated with diarrhea, allergy, and obesity. The African children had lots of species associated with leanness and also much higher levels of beneficial short-chain fatty acids that protect against inflammation, highlighting the connection between what you eat in childhood and developing a host of ailments later on. Seen through this lens, getting our kids (and ourselves) to eat more plants takes on epic importance.

The feeding-frenzy effect is important to keep in mind if you're following a low-carb diet but eating mostly animal protein high in fat, and it's why my Live Dirty, Eat Clean Plan, which incorporates fiber-rich foods like legumes, is so successful at rehabbing the microbiome.

Are You Forgetting to Eat Fiber?

Not enough fiber can be even worse for your microbiome than too much sugar, starch, and fat. Most Americans only eat about half the recommended 25 to 35 grams of fiber daily, and much of it in processed, less beneficial forms. Certain types of dietary fiber are what we call prebiotics: non-digestible ingredients that encourage the growth of beneficial species and are a crucial part of restoring and maintaining microbial balance. Foods like lentils, beans, oats, apples, nuts, and flaxseeds increase the population of helpful *Lactobacillus* species in the gut, while insufficient dietary fiber has a negative effect on both the amount and diversity of gut bacteria—something we'll discuss in more detail in Chapter 9.

Are Your Bacteria Intoxicated?

A glass or two of red wine may be good for your heart but not for your microbiome. Studies show that just one drink per day in women and two in men can induce dysbiosis and bacterial overgrowth. Levels of good bacteria like *Lactobacillus* fall, while potential pathogens rise, leading to an increase in toxins and other chemicals that can cause inflammation, damage the liver, and increase permeability of the gut. Most of the overgrowth happens in the small intestine and can lead to malnourishment because the excess bacteria consume the nutrients that the small intestine would normally absorb. Some studies report an incidence of small intestinal bacterial overgrowth (SIBO) in alcoholics that's three times that of the general population.

Detecting Dysbiosis: Are Your Bacteria as Stressed Out as You Are?

Stress isn't just bad for you; it's bad for your gut bacteria, too. A study from Ohio State University showed that stress affects the amount of mucus production in the stomach, which changes the composition, diversity, and amount of gut bacteria growing in your gut. Not only is there less species variation with stress, but the numbers of potentially harmful bacteria rise, too, which increases our susceptibility to infection. It's why when we're run down, tired, and stressed, we're more likely to get sick.

In my gastroenterology practice, mind-body relaxation techniques like biofeedback, which incorporates guided meditation, visual imagery, and deep breathing, are a crucial part of rehabbing the microbiome and achieving digestive wellness, and we've found them to be successful across a wide spectrum of GI disorders.

Detecting Dysbiosis: Have You Had Any Major Infections?

Antibiotics aren't the only cause of dysbiosis. Gastrointestinal infections themselves can deplete the microbiome, and the subsequent decrease in microbial richness can lead to increased susceptibility to disease. Many patients trace the beginnings of their decline in health to an infectious event—from Montezuma's revenge in Mexico to dysentery on safari in southern Africa to a bout of giardia from contaminated water closer to home. Post-infectious irritable bowel syndrome is a well-described phenomenon, and up to 10 percent of patients with inflammatory bowel disease like Crohn's and ulcerative colitis point to a significant infectious event that marks the beginning of their illness, particularly if their microbiome was already compromised from prior antibiotic use.

Many Roads Can Lead to Dysbiosis

Most of the patients I see with dysbiosis have multiple risk factors, including treatment with acid-suppressing drugs, lots of antibiotics, intermittent steroid use for inflammation, and a steady diet of junk food in their early years. Taking antibiotics for acne tends to be the most damaging factor because those drugs are so effective against gut bacteria and the treatment usually lasts months or even years—but usually it's a combination of different causes that tips people over the edge and creates symptoms. And the symptoms, which are really the clinical manifestation of dysbiosis, vary tremendously from person to person.

Some people get frequent vaginal yeast infections; others have bloating or GI distress; some develop hair loss, acne, or unexplained hives. Extreme fatigue may be the only symptom, while others just complain of feeling "off" without really being able to qualify it further. I suspect that the symptoms one develops are closely linked to which species of bacteria are depleted or dominant, but we lack large population-based studies that correlate specific risk factors with symptoms.

Autoimmune disease—conditions such as Crohn's disease, thyroiditis, lupus, multiple sclerosis (MS), celiac disease, and dozens of others—can be a sign of dysbiosis, and one that's increasingly common, affecting one in five Americans. While it's important to remember that dysbiosis isn't the only cause of autoimmune diseases or the other conditions I describe in this chapter, being familiar with the wide range of potential manifestations can help you figure out if damage to your microbiome could be at the root of your health problems.

Less Is Often More: Chelsea's Story

Chelsea was diagnosed with MS in her early thirties. In the five years since her diagnosis she'd been taking steroids and a monoclonal antibody therapy known to cause a lethal viral infection of the brain similar to mad cow disease. Both drugs had weakened her immune system and put her at high risk for urinary tract infections (UTIs), of which she'd had several, each necessitating weeks of antibiotics. She was also taking an acid-suppressing medication in the form of a proton pump inhibitor to counteract stomach irritation from the steroids.

When Chelsea arrived at my office for her first appointment, she'd been doing the SAD GAS diet from my book *Gutbliss* for a few weeks: no soy, artificial sweeteners, dairy, gluten, alcohol, or sugar. Although this regimen had reduced her bloating quite a bit, she was still having foul-smelling gas, loose and irregular bowel movements, abdominal cramping, and severe fatigue. It was hard to know how much of her fatigue was related to MS, but Chelsea's other symptoms were consistent with dysbiosis, and it was telling that they had gotten more severe after several rounds of antibiotics the previous year.

Tackling Chelsea's dysbiosis was challenging because the medications she was taking were a contributing factor, but they couldn't easily be discontinued. The side effects of the monoclonal antibody were potentially fatal, but rare, and less deleterious to her microbes than the combination of steroids and antibiotics, so we decided to leave that drug in place. It took us several months to wean her off the steroids, but once we did, the frequent UTIs stopped, as did the need for antibiotics, and she didn't need the proton pump inhibitor to counteract the effects of the steroids anymore.

The next step was to go all the way with her diet, cutting out almost all processed foods, especially grains, and really ramping up the green leafy vegetables—strategies that Terry Wahls, MD, advocates for MS in *The Wahls Protocol* and that also work wonders for the microbiome. Chelsea was also on a prescription-strength probiotic. Two years into this regimen, we're finally seeing results: Chelsea's GI symptoms are significantly better, and her MS and fatigue have improved, too, despite her being on less medication!

Conditions Associated with Dysbiosis

Because we know that microbes are integrally involved in most of our bodily functions, it shouldn't come as a surprise that microbial imbalance is turning out to be the driving force behind many of our new and existing disorders. Virtually every week there's new evidence linking it to a medical condition. Some, like leaky gut, are relatively new maladies, while others, like depression, have been around for hundreds of years but are now reaching epidemic proportions, mirroring our modern era's high rates of dysbiosis.

The following conditions are the ones I see most commonly in my

TABLE 5–2 • Dysbiosis May Be the Root
Cause of the Following Conditions

- Food cravings
- Bloating
- Weight gain
- Yeast overgrowth
- Irritable bowel syndrome (IBS)
- Inflammatory bowel disease (IBD)
- Small intestinal bacterial overgrowth (SIBO)
- Leaky gut
- Parasites
- Celiac/gluten sensitivity
- Vaginosis
- Food allergies and sensitivities
- Chronic fatigue syndrome (CFS)
- Depression
- Skin conditions (acne, rosacea, eczema)

office in people with dysbiosis. While alterations in the microbiome aren't the only cause, dysbiosis often plays a central role, and rebalancing gut microbes frequently leads to a significant improvement in symptoms.

"My Microbes Made Me Do It": Food Cravings

As I mentioned in the Introduction, microbial cells outnumber our own cells ten to one, making us more microbe than human in some unexpected ways. Food cravings, anxiety, memory, mood, and how easily we lose or gain weight are just some of the traits that are heavily influenced by our gut bacteria. The article "Is Eating Behavior Manipulated by the Gastrointestinal Microbiota?: Evolutionary Pressures and Potential Mechanisms," published in the October 2014 issue of the journal *BioEssays*, raised the provocative idea that our bacteria may indeed be running the show—controlling our thoughts and deeds in order to ensure their own survival!

We often blame our food cravings on our lack of willpower. It turns out that our microbes might have something to do with it. When sugar-loving species gain a foothold in our gut, we may find ourselves craving (and eating) more sweets. What we think of as just a wicked sweet tooth may actually represent specific communities of bacteria directing us to behave in a way that ensures their survival, despite its negative effect on our own health. Gut bacteria are able to influence our food choices by releasing molecules that affect our brain, including hormones like serotonin that affect mood and make us feel good after eating certain foods. They can even change the properties of taste receptors so that particular flavors are more or less satisfying to our palate.

There's intense competition for space within the digestive tract, so microbes are under a lot of selective pressure to procure the right food to enhance their survival—or suppress their competitors'. As Carlo Maley, PhD, one of the authors of the *BioEssays* article, describes it: "From the microbe's perspective, what we eat is a matter of life and death." That explains why so many of us feel powerless to resist certain kinds of food—we may not actually be the ones making the decision!

I've observed this phenomenon repeatedly in patients with dysbiosis. Strong sugar or carbohydrate cravings are almost always part of the symptom complex—and one of the first things to improve after rebalancing their microbiome. It also explains why people on a low-carb regimen have reduced cravings for sugary, starchy foods within a week or so of eliminating them from their diet: they're also reducing the species that thrive on those foods, since the food we eat determines what sort of bacteria we grow in our gut garden.

Bloating

There are lots of things that can bloat you (I wrote a whole book about it!), but dysbiosis is definitely at the top of the list. Microbial imbalance leads to overproduction of bloat-causing hydrogen and methane gases, along with attendant abdominal discomfort, a change in bowel habits, smelly gas, a strange odor to stool, or explosive bowel movements. Any or all of these, whether as constant problems or as symptoms that ebb and flow throughout the week, may be signals that all is not well in your microbiome.

Eliminating my SAD GAS foods (soy, artificial sweeteners, dairy, gluten, alcohol, and sugar) is helpful, but some forms of bloating require serious dietary changes as well as repopulation with healthy microbes. I'll explain the art and science of how we accomplish this in Chapter 12, "Bugs over Drugs: Probiotics and Other Supplements."

Weight Gain

We can predict obesity with 90 percent accuracy just by examining your gut bacteria, and we can make skinny mice fat by inoculating them with microbes from obese mice. Studies show that overweight mice can actually extract more calories than their normal-sized peers from exactly the same food. We see the same phenomenon in humans: if your gut bacteria are out of whack, you may be packing on the pounds despite eating a diet identical to that of someone who's not gaining weight.

When we view weight gain through the lens of an altered microbiome, it explains the skyrocketing rates of obesity that parallel our widespread use of antibiotics. A high-fat, high-sugar, nutrient-poor diet is also clearly a risk factor, although the food itself may not be the direct cause of obesity but rather the secondary factor that induces the microbial changes that make us gain weight. We'll explore the fascinating link between our microbes and our weight in Chapter 6, "Are Our Bacteria Making Us Fat?"

Yeast Overgrowth

Yeasts are single-celled organisms that are part of the fungi family. They multiply by budding—splitting off in bulges from the parent cell wall—which can be especially rapid (within a couple of hours) when there's lots of starchy, sugary food around. The sugars in these foods are consumed (fermented) by yeast and converted to alcohol and carbon dioxide—which is why yeast has been used by humans for centuries for making products like bread, wine, and beer.

We all have yeast in our body—yeast cells are present in low levels in the human colon, where they help with digestion. It's when yeast-like candida and other fungi grow too rapidly that we have a problem. This form of dysbiosis is especially common after taking antibiotics, which causes a reduction in essential bacteria and allows yeast to proliferate unchecked and colonize moist parts of the body. Yeast overgrowth can show up as a cheesy white vaginal discharge; thick white patches on the tongue or in the mouth; red areas under the breasts, between the toes, in the ears, or around the anus that look like diaper rash; dandruff on the scalp; pustules in the groin or armpits; or nail bed infec-

---

TABLE 5–3 • Symptoms of Yeast Overgrowth

- Bloating
- Constipation
- Depression
- Diarrhea
- Fatigue
- Food sensitivities
- Headaches
- Impaired concentration
- Irritability
- Nail infections
- Oral thrush (white lesions in mouth)
- Poor memory
- Rectal itching
- Skin problems (eczema, acne, hives, athlete's foot, ringworm, dandruff)
- Sugar/carbohydrate cravings
- Unstable blood sugar
- Vaginal itching

tions. And the symptoms vary tremendously, too, from GI complaints to fatigue, mood disorders, and even depression.

People usually want to treat their yeast problem with aggressive over-the-counter or prescription antifungals, but repopulating the gut with essential bacteria that can crowd out yeast and keep their growth in check is the hallmark of a successful treatment program, not just temporarily suppressing them with medication.

Reduction Without Restoration: Olivia's Story

Olivia was a gaunt, ill-appearing thirty-nine-year-old woman who came to see me for bloating, gas, and concerns about yeast overgrowth. A year earlier, she had developed a severe vaginal yeast infection after being treated for pneumonia with two months of antibiotics. She was doing phone consultations with a doctor who billed himself as a yeast specialist who had prescribed eight weeks of fluconazole, an antifungal with potential side effects of liver disease and cardiac arrhythmias. When her yeast infection still wasn't resolved, he recommended an additional eight weeks of therapy. Since the onset of the yeast infection she had been on a strict diet with no grains whatsoever, no fruit, no starchy vegetables, and no sugar, honey, or sweeteners of any kind. She didn't enjoy vegetables, so she had literally been eating nothing but meat, chicken, and eggs for the last year.

I assured Olivia that, after all that therapy and the rigid diet, there were probably no yeast alive anywhere in her body and that her bloating and gas were likely the result of insufficient quantities of essential bacteria rather than yeast overgrowth. She was fervent in her belief that yeast were still invading her body and needed to be treated, and it took multiple conversations with me and my nutritionist and a blood test that showed normal levels of antibodies to candida to convince her otherwise.

Getting Olivia to stop the fluconazole was easy, but persuading her to liberalize her diet was much more challenging. She was starving herself and her microbiome. She and her bacteria desperately needed some real food and nutrients. Eventually, because she felt so poorly, Olivia relented and started to add in first small amounts of lentils and zucchini, then green beans and carrots, and finally some less sugary fruits like Granny Smith apples and berries. Our nutritionist persuaded her to eat quinoa a couple of times, but she was so afraid of anything that contained carbohydrates that she would only eat a few teaspoons. Still, over the next year, with the help of a lot of nutrition coaching, some therapy, and a good probiotic, Olivia gradually gained some weight back and started to feel better.

Yeast overgrowth is a real phenomenon, and one that conventional doctors are often skeptical and poorly informed about. But yeast paranoia is also a real problem, and sometimes people have to be discouraged from adopting a too severe diet that isn't nourishing to their good gut microbes, or from overtreating for something that's not actually a problem anymore. Stepping back and giving your body time to heal is sometimes the best approach, especially if you've vanquished the offending agents and are working to restore your microbes with nourishing food, a good probiotic, and sufficient rest.

Irritable Bowel Syndrome (IBS)

We tend to lump everyone with a digestive complaint together under the IBS umbrella. By definition, IBS is a diagnosis of exclusion, another way of saying, "you feel crummy, but everything looks fine." But anyone suffering from IBS will tell you that things are definitely not fine, regardless of how normal their colonoscopy, endoscopy, or labs may appear.

Part of the problem is that we've been looking for explanations we can see with the naked eye, when the cause, at least for some IBS sufferers, is microscopic. Several studies show changes in the bacterial composition of the stool in patients with IBS. Diarrhea-predominant IBS tends to be associated with lower-than-normal levels of *Bifidobac-*

terium and *Lactobacillus*, while constipation-predominant IBS has higher-than-normal levels of *Veillonella* species.

As many as one-third of patients with IBS develop symptoms after an acute infectious event like traveler's diarrhea or food poisoning—what we sometimes refer to as post-infectious IBS. It's especially common after infections with bacteria such as *Campylobacter*, *Salmonella*, and *Shigella*, or with parasites such as giardia, although it's unclear if it's the actual infection that causes the symptoms or the microbial imbalance that develops afterward. An acute infection can crowd out good bacteria as the population of pathogens grows exponentially, and even after the rogue organism is curtailed, the ratio of good to bad microbes may still be askew. Microbes may even be involved in how bad IBS makes us feel: perturbations in gut bacteria in mice can affect how pain is perceived, leading to the visceral hypersensitivity that's typical of IBS.

The conventional treatment approach is to alleviate symptoms using prescription drugs, not unearth and remediate the underlying cause. Most of the medications—including the psychiatric drugs that are frequently prescribed—have lots of side effects and aren't particularly effective. The finding of alterations in the microbiome as a major contributor to IBS offers exciting promise for new ways to address symptoms through restoration of microbial balance.

When Bugs Work Better Than Drugs

Monica had been diagnosed with IBS as a freshman in college, when the combination of lots of stress and poor eating habits led to her spending lots of time in the bathroom. Like many of us, she also had a history of frequent antibiotics in childhood for ear infections. Monica had urgency and frequent loose bowel movements every morning, which sometimes made her late for class or caused her to miss it altogether. She developed anxiety around not having immediate access to a bathroom, and her social life suffered as she became more withdrawn and isolated.

She was prescribed a potent antidiarrheal agent, which took care of the urgency and loose stools but gave her cramping and constipation, so she wasn't keen to use it other than for emergency situations when she didn't have good bathroom access. Several different types of antidepressant drugs were recommended and tried, but all of them had side effects that were almost as intolerable as her GI symptoms. One made her extraordinarily tired, another gave her dry mouth and affected her vision, and the last two she tried caused significant weight gain.

Monica was resigned to living with her bathroom issues when a friend suggested she try a probiotic. She bought the first one she saw at the pharmacy and noticed an almost immediate improvement the first week, but by the end of the second week her symptoms were back to their not so great baseline. She tried several more probiotics over the next few months and had fleeting glimmers of improvement here and there, but her symptoms always came back after a few weeks.

When I saw Monica in consultation, I recommended a much stronger probiotic with additional bacterial strains and told her she should commit to taking it for several months before deciding it wasn't helping. I also had her add a lot more plant fiber into her diet. She was skeptical but agreed to give it a try, and within about three months she was seeing light at the end of the tunnel. Eight months later she was down to two formed stools a day, with good control, no urgency, and no abdominal pain—an acceptable baseline that the prescription drugs weren't able to achieve.

Inflammatory Bowel Disease (IBD)

We learned in Chapter 3 that not enough childhood exposure to germs, lots of antibiotics, plus the Western diet high in fat, starch, and sugar are all risk factors for developing Crohn's and ulcerative colitis, the two forms of IBD. In studies, people with IBD can be differentiated from healthy individuals by evaluating the bacteria present in their stool, and different types of Crohn's disease are associated with different microbial changes—further evidence that the microbiome plays a key role in these diseases.

In my gastroenterology practice, a plant-based diet low in processed carbohydrates and refined sugar, in combination with high-dose prescription-strength probiotics, has been extraordinarily successful for getting IBD into remission and reducing or eliminating the need for toxic medications.

Small Intestinal Bacterial Overgrowth (SIBO)

The small intestine is hardly sterile, but it typically has a lot less bacteria than the colon, the main living quarters for gut bacteria. SIBO is really just another term for dysbiosis that occurs when large amounts of not-so-good bacteria take up residence in the small intestine, causing gas, bloating, abdominal discomfort, and sometimes diarrhea or constipation. Nutritional deficiencies can also be part of the clinical presentation, as gut bacteria may affect absorption of nutrients or consume them themselves. Antibiotic use is a major cause of SIBO, but impaired bowel motility and partial bowel obstruction that result in stasis (i.e., slowing down or stopping the movement) of intestinal contents, and acid suppression that creates a hospitable environment for bacteria to overgrow, are also risk factors.

We can test for SIBO by administering a poorly absorbed sugar by mouth that gets fermented by gut bacteria in the intestines. High levels of bacteria produce greater-than-expected levels of methane and hydrogen gases, which are expelled through the lungs and measured in the breath (via a lactulose or hydrogen breath test). Although breath tests can be useful, I don't find them to be very reliable, so I tend to rely more on a clinical diagnosis based on history, physical exam, and signs and symptoms.

TABLE 5–4 • Symptoms of SIBO

- Abdominal pain/cramping
- Bloating
- Constipation
- Depression
- Diarrhea
- Excessive gas
- Fatigue
- Food cravings
- Headaches
- Rashes

Some physicians treat SIBO with an oral antibiotic called rifaximin, also known as Xifaxan. The theory is that because rifaximin has activity against a broad spectrum of bacteria that are overgrowing in the small intestine, using it to reduce their populations should lead to an improvement in symptoms. And it frequently does. The problem, of course, is that rifaximin, like all antibiotics, also has activity against essential bacteria and diminishes those populations, too. The result is usually an initial amelioration followed by relapse a few months later.

Too Many Drugs—Not Enough Bugs

My friend is a dermatologist who, like many of our colleagues, believes wholeheartedly in the benefits of pharmaceutical intervention. Last year her husband developed a *Salmonella* infection with diarrhea and abdominal cramping. He felt crummy but didn't have any of the indications for treatment with antibiotics, such as severe diarrhea, a high fever, or *Salmonella* growing in the blood, nor was he elderly, immunocompromised, or in any way at risk for developing more severe illness. Yet despite medical guidelines that recommend only oral hydration or IV fluids, she decided to treat him with an antibiotic, Ciprofloxacin, "just in case."

Treating uncomplicated *Salmonella* with antibiotics actually prolongs the carrier state—the amount of time you may be excreting the bacteria in your stool and be in danger of infecting others—without doing anything to shorten or improve the course of the illness. When he wasn't showing improvement after about five days, my friend decided to add more antibiotics and prescribed Bactrim and Levaquin. All told, her husband was on antibiotics for three weeks for a condition that requires no antibiotic therapy at all. He eventually made a good recovery and after a month was feeling back to baseline.

Her husband had a history of reflux and had been on omeprazole for years, a proton pump inhibitor that suppresses stomach acid production. These drugs increase the risk of getting gastroenteritis because of the reduction in acid, which, when present in normal amounts, can kill invading bacteria such as *Salmonella*. A few months after the acute event, he started to complain about severe bloating, burping, and abdominal pain. His wife was convinced that this meant his acid reflux was worse, so she doubled his dose of proton pump inhibitor and added more anti-acid therapy in the form of an H2 blocker at night. His symptoms continued, although the severe distention, tenderness, and cramping were centered around his navel—the wrong location for acid reflux, which usually causes discomfort in the chest, just under the sternum.

At this point she began to worry that the *Salmonella* had recurred, but extensive stool testing and blood cultures were negative, and he was having only minor episodes of diarrhea. His wife wanted to give him more antibiotics but was persuaded not to. His symptoms and the time frame were classic for SIBO (onset following a severe GI infection, in the setting of antibiotics and acid-suppressing drugs), but I knew my friend would need definitive proof, so we arranged for a hydrogen breath test, which was markedly positive. We stopped his acid suppression medication, added a probiotic, and made a few changes to his diet. He eventually got better, but it took about six months, and during that time there was a lot of pressure to continue treating him with more drugs—antacids, antibiotics, a pro-motility agent to help move the bacteria through the small intestine. "There must be something we can prescribe to fix this," was her constant thought.

Sometimes more access to medical therapy isn't such a good thing, especially when the effects on your microbiome are cumulative, as they are with acid-blocking medicines and antibiotics. It's important to take a step back and ask yourself whether the drugs you're taking could in some way be contributing to your problem—a challenging but essential step when you don't seem to be getting better. Pharmaceutical cures can be lifesaving, but watchful waiting while you allow your body—and your microbes—to heal and recover is sometimes the most judicious approach.

Leaky Gut

Your digestive tract forms a hollow tube that runs from your mouth to your anus. Your intestinal contents aren't really inside your body until they're absorbed through the lining of that tube into your bloodstream. This inner lining forms a selective barrier that allows some substances to pass through while preventing others. Bacterial imbalance and overgrowth of potentially harmful microbes can compromise the integrity of the barrier, allowing toxins and other undesirables to enter and interfering with absorption of nutrients—a condition called leaky gut.

Overgrowth of yeast species, such as candida, and parasitic infection have been implicated in the development of leaky gut, but a diet high in refined sugar, processed food, preservatives, and chemicals are contributing factors, as is consumption of gluten, a protein found in wheat, rye, and barley that we'll discuss in depth later in this chapter. Too much alcohol, radiation treatment, and chemotherapy can all damage the gut lining, and chronic stress can weaken your immune system, affecting your ability to fight off invading pathogens and worsening the symptoms of leaky gut. Medications such as aspirin and NSAIDs damage the lining of your gut, antacids change the pH, and steroids alter the intestinal milieu—and all are associated with increased intestinal permeability (IP).

It's helpful to think of leaky gut more as a mechanism than a disease, since there's such a wide range of signs and symptoms associated with it. It's a precondition for developing autoimmune disease, since it's the increase in intestinal permeability—the opening of the door from our gut into our body—that allows toxins to enter and then trigger an immune response. Leaky gut has also been implicated in food allergies, GI distress, and a host of nonspecific complaints, including headaches, hair loss, fatigue, joint pain, rashes, hives, brain fog, memory loss, and increased susceptibility to infection. Mainstream medicine is only now beginning to recognize leaky gut as a legitimate condition, despite the fact that it's an incredibly common problem, reflecting the high rates of microbial discord at its root.

Like many manifestations of dysbiosis, leaky gut is primarily a clinical diagnosis, although I sometimes perform an intestinal permeability (IP) test to assess the integrity of the gut lining. It involves drinking two sugar solutions: mannitol is a small sugar that should normally pass easily through the lining and be detectable in high amounts in the urine, while lactulose is a larger sugar that has difficulty passing through an intact membrane and should therefore be present in much smaller amounts. The ratio of lactulose to mannitol is what helps us assess whether or not permeability is increased. Many patients ask for "the leaky gut test," but it's important to be aware that the IP test is affected by other factors (extreme exercise, for example), can easily revert to normal after a few weeks if you've been following a strict diet or taking probiotics, and is simply a test that measures permeability—not one that on its own confirms or negates a diagnosis of leaky gut.

Risk Factors and an Acute Event

Hilary didn't have a history of lots of antibiotic use in the past, but she was a picky eater in childhood who avoided fruits and vegetables like the plague. She was now in her thirties and in good health until a case of severe gastroenteritis with nausea, vomiting, fever, and dehydration led to a five-day hospitalization. The cause of the gastroenteritis was never identified, but because she had a fever she was treated with two different intravenous antibiotics while in the hospital and discharged on an additional ten-day course of oral antibiotics.

Hilary felt better by the time she completed the antibiotics, but three months after the hospitalization she developed severe bloating and mushy stool that she described as having an oatmeal consistency. Upper endoscopy and colonoscopy were unrevealing, and biopsies were negative for celiac disease or any other abnormalities. A month later she was prescribed an antibiotic for a UTI, and then another one for a sinus infection. The mushy stool got worse and she developed rosacea, vaginal yeast infections, and headaches. An IP test was eventually ordered and was positive.

Although Hilary hadn't taken a lot of antibiotics before her hospitalization, she had been on acid suppressive therapy for years for symptoms of acid reflux and had a long history of daily ibuprofen use for various aches and pains—both major risk factors for developing increased intestinal permeability. The acute gastroenteritis and the antibiotics that followed were likely the inciting events that led to the abnormal stools, bloating, rosacea, yeast infections, and headaches—all manifestations of leaky gut. Her symptoms eventually resolved after several months of dietary therapy, probiotics, and discontinuation of the ibuprofen and acid blockers.

Hilary's experience highlights the importance of how a background of risk factors that you may not even be aware of can increase your likelihood of developing leaky gut after an acute event like an infection, or a course of antibiotics.

Parasites

Many of the patients I see with GI symptoms like gas and bloating or a change in bowel habits are concerned that they may have a parasite. And many of them do: the Centers for Disease Control and Prevention (CDC) estimates that almost one-third of us harbor parasites, even those who have never traveled far from home. That may be surprising to you, but humans and parasites have a long association: medical anthropologists have pointed out that our ancestors were covered with parasites, and that chronic exposure to these organisms helped their immune systems develop tolerance—something that confers important benefits later on. The key question for patients who come to see me with concerns about parasites is not whether or not they have one but whether that is actually what's causing their GI symptoms.

Overwhelming parasitic infestation can cause dysbiosis by crowding out essential bacteria and can also lead to leaky gut if the parasites take root in the lining of the digestive tract and compromise the barrier function.

We're not sure whether parasites like *Blastocystis hominis*, an intestinal protozoa found worldwide, is a true pathogen that causes symptoms or a harmless commensal—a freeloading tenant, one might say, but not a dangerous one—that's just an innocent bystander. Part of the challenge is that some people who have *Blastocystis* report feeling better when the *Blastocystis* is treated, while others don't. But treatment isn't always a good idea for some of these hard-to-categorize parasites because the antiparasitic agents frequently have antibacterial effects and, if taken often enough, can wipe out a lot of essential bacteria and worsen dysbiosis.

If there really seems to be no other explanation for the GI symptoms other than *Blastocystis*, I'll usually treat it, but I try to avoid standard therapy such as the antibiotic metronidazole in favor of a more holistic approach using probiotics such as *Saccharomyces boulardii* for eradication.

Infections with parasites such as giardia can lead to nausea, diarrhea, bloating, and even IBS, but as we explored in Chapter 3, some studies have suggested that other parasites, especially helminths such as hookworm, can be an effective therapy for Crohn's disease and other illnesses that involve a heightened immune response by dampening the immune system and improving symptoms.

TABLE 5–5 • Nonpathogenic Intestinal Protozoa

- *Chilomastix mesnili*
- *Endolimax nana*
- *Entamoeba coli*
- *Entamoeba dispar*
- *Entamoeba hartmanni*
- *Entamoeba polecki*
- *Iodamoeba bütschlii*

Nonpathogenic intestinal protozoa are parasites that can inhabit the digestive tract but aren't associated with illness. They're not felt to be harmful, even in people with weak immune systems, so people who have these protozoa in their stool should be evaluated for other causes of their symptoms, although their presence may be a sign of dysbiosis.

Celiac Disease and Gluten Sensitivity

Celiac disease is an autoimmune disorder that damages the lining of the small intestine as a result of eating gluten, a protein found in wheat, rye, and barley. People with celiac disease can have a wide variety of nonspecific symptoms or occasionally be completely asymptomatic. Gluten sensitivity, also known as gluten intolerance, can lead to similar symptoms, but it isn't considered an autoimmune disorder, and there's no damage to the lining of the small intestine when we take biopsies of it and examine them under the microscope, the way there is with celiac disease. Gluten sensitivity may represent a halfway point between normal GI function and celiac disease; in some people, it may be a precursor for developing celiac disease.

Although you may think of gluten-free diets (GFDs) as a recent fad, the foundation for our intolerance to gluten was laid down over ten thousand years ago when our nomadic hunter-gatherer ancestors began to domesticate crops, introducing gluten into the diet for the first time. Since then, wheat has been hybridized and crossbred to increase the yield and decrease production costs, and high-yield dwarf triticum wheat now represents virtually all of the wheat consumed worldwide.

About a third of people of European ancestry carry genes that predispose them to developing celiac disease, but only a small percentage actually develop the disease, proving that genes are necessary but not sufficient for causing it. There seems to be some sort of trigger that tells the immune system whether to treat gluten as food or as a foreign substance it should react to. We didn't know what that trigger was, but several studies now point to alterations in the microbiome as the culprit.

Breast-feeding is protective against developing autoimmune diseases in general, and studies have now shown that it specifically helps protect against the development of celiac disease. Breast-fed children have more *Bifidobacteria* than their formula-fed peers (which help dampen the body's response to inflammation), and children with celiac disease have lower-than-normal levels of *Bifidobacteria* and higher levels of *E. coli* and other less desirable species (which amplify inflammation and can cause leaky gut). Researcher Alessio Fasano, MD, considers leaky gut to be at the heart of why people develop celiac disease. It's the open door that allows gluten to enter the body and run amok.

Studies have now also confirmed an astounding association between antibiotic use and the development of celiac disease that may explain why dysbiosis responds so well to the elimination of gluten from the diet. People with new-onset celiac disease are 40 percent more likely to have been prescribed antibiotics shortly before diagnosis than their healthy peers, and the risk increases the more antibiotics you're prescribed. Many of the patients in my practice develop celiac disease or gluten sensitivity after being treated with metronidazole, a drug with high affinity for destroying gut bacteria, although virtually any antibiotic seems capable of inducing an intolerance to gluten by altering the microbial content of the gut and increasing the permeability of the lining.

Researchers from Finland reported that GI symptoms may persist in patients with celiac disease even after years of following a GFD because of ongoing abnormalities in their microbiome. These microbe-associated symptoms may still be present even after small bowel mucosal changes and blood work have normalized, so going gluten free may not be enough—if you have celiac disease, repopulating your microbiome may also be an important part of getting your symptoms under control.

Unmasking Disease

Mary had been treated with two courses of metronidazole after a bout of food poisoning. Most of these episodes are self-limited and don't require any medication, but because she had lingering symptoms of nausea and diarrhea, her doctor prescribed antibiotics. Three months later she was treated with doxycycline for the possibility of Lyme disease after a summer in the Berkshires. The usual testing for Lyme was negative, but she had found a tick on her leg and was concerned, so she requested antibiotic therapy. A checkup with her doctor six weeks later revealed new-onset iron deficiency anemia, and she continued to have diarrhea, which was now accompanied by bloating and weight loss. Suspecting another infection, her internist treated her with two more courses of antibiotics, despite negative cultures, blood work, and stool studies. All told, she received about eight weeks of antibiotic therapy.

I was asked to evaluate her and exclude blood loss from the GI tract as a possible cause of the anemia. Her colonoscopy was unremarkable, and upper endoscopy revealed a normal esophagus, stomach, and duodenum. But biopsies from the duodenum (the first part of the small intestine) showed changes suggestive of early celiac disease—mild blunting of the fingerlike projections in the small intestine known as villi, and an increase in the amount of inflammatory white blood cells (lymphocytes) found in the lining—a sign of the body's response to inflammation. Blood tests showed positive antibodies and a genetic profile that put her in a high-risk category for developing celiac disease.

Mary was not happy when I discussed the results of the endoscopy and the blood tests with her. She believed that her symptoms were all the result of an infection and that more antibiotics would eventually solve the problem. There was definitely skepticism when I explained that the large amounts of antibiotics she'd received were probably responsible for her developing celiac disease. The blood tests indicated a genetic susceptibility, and the virus that caused her food poisoning may have crowded out some of her essential bacterial species, but the antibiotics were the nail that sealed her gluten-free coffin.

She reluctantly agreed to try a GFD, but after a month there was no improvement in her symptoms. We asked her to keep a two-week food journal, which revealed an enormous amount of gluten-free processed carbohydrates such as cookies, pancakes, bread, and pasta. I asked her to avoid anything with a gluten-free label on it, and our nutrition coach did a few supermarket trips with her and created some easy-to-follow meal plans. But there was still the issue of her depleted microbiome. Mary was the consummate picky eater, so it took some convincing to get her to increase her intake of high-fiber foods and green leafy vegetables—blending them in a green smoothie with some berries and coconut water was her preferred way of getting them down. I started her on a prescription-strength high-dose probiotic that she added to the smoothie after blending. It took a while, but after about six months she was finally feeling back to normal—still missing her bread and pasta, but adhering pretty closely to the new diet and enjoying her good health.

Because Mary had evidence of celiac disease on endoscopy and wasn't just gluten sensitive, my recommendation was that she stay on a strict GFD. It's unclear whether people who develop gluten sensitivity as a manifestation of dysbiosis after antibiotics ever regain their toler-

TABLE 5-6 • Signs and Symptoms
Associated with Celiac Disease

- Abdominal pain
- Arthritis
- Bloating
- Brain fog
- Constipation
- Depression
- Diarrhea
- Fatigue
- Gas
- Gastrointestinal bleeding
- Hair loss
- Infertility
- Iron deficiency
- Mouth sores
- Muscle weakness
- Nausea
- Neuropathy
- Osteoporosis
- Rashes (dermatitis herpetiformis)
- Vitamin deficiencies
- Vomiting
- Weight gain
- Weight loss

ance, but given the nature of today's wheat, which releases more glucose into your bloodstream than table sugar, plus the fact that it doesn't have much nutritional value, quitting it for good seems like the most advisable option.

Vaginosis

Bacterial imbalance doesn't just occur in your gut. It can happen in your vagina, too, leading to a condition called bacterial vaginosis, or BV. Vaginal yeast infections after antibiotics are a type of dysbiosis, and so is BV. When the normal vaginal flora is altered as a result of antibiotic use, douching, or a change in pH, essential *Lactobacillus* species that normally repel other species by producing acid may be reduced, leading to overgrowth of a wide variety of bacteria that can run amok in the vagina. Lots of different species have been associated with BV, including *Gardnerella, Prevotella, Mycoplasma, Mobiluncus, Bacte-*

roides, and *Peptostreptococcus*. The decrease in protective *Lactobacillus* species also leads to increased susceptibility to UTIs, sexually transmitted diseases (including HIV, human immunodeficiency virus), the development of pelvic inflammatory disease (which can lead to infertility), and miscarriages. This "low *Lactobacillus* state" that defines BV can also enhance the spread of sexually transmitted diseases because having fewer *Lactobacillus* species around allows viral replication and shedding to proceed unchecked.

The vaginal discharge characteristic of BV is off-white and not as thick or itchy as that of a yeast infection, although it can have a similar fishy odor. If you've been diagnosed with BV, it's important to consider not reaching for an oral or topical antibiotic such as metronidazole—the therapy of choice in most gynecology practices—because while it will curtail the growth of the less desirable species, it will also further reduce the healthy bacterial population, leading to a vicious cycle of recurrence. As in most manifestations of dysbiosis, repopulation of healthy bacteria is the key. In addition to dietary changes, I frequently recommend taking probiotics that contain high levels of *Lactobacillus* orally as well as inserting them vaginally to treat BV.

Food Allergies and Sensitivities

Food allergies and sensitivities have reached alarmingly high rates, affecting fifteen million Americans. On average, about two children in every classroom have food allergies, many of them severe or life-threatening. Wiping out gut bacteria leads to food allergies in mice, and the same seems to be true in humans, where we can trace a direct relationship between the widespread use of antibiotics, especially in children, and skyrocketing rates of food allergies. Replenishing gut bacteria in mice, particularly with *Clostridia* and *Bacteroides* species, seems to ameliorate many of the allergies, although it's unclear whether that same degree of reversibility is possible in humans, especially when species are eliminated early in life.

Food sensitivities and intolerances can't easily be tested for because blood and skin tests that measure immune responses usually fail to detect them. Even testing for full-blown food allergies can be unwieldy, with people sometimes testing positive for allergies to multiple foods that they eat every day without any problem, or not reacting to anything on the panel despite documented reactions. Many of the patients I see come in with reams of tests showing long lists of foods they "can't" eat, or they themselves have crossed most foods off their list because of possible reactions.

While reactions to specific foods are possible and common, for many people their overreactive immune system is a result of dysbiosis-induced leaky gut. When the gut lining is damaged, large undigested food particles that normally would be kept in the gut can leak through, entering the bloodstream and eliciting an allergic immune response. That's why the big-picture approach to food sensitivities is to rehab the microbiome, not just to create longer and longer lists of what you can't eat.

Chronic Fatigue Syndrome (CFS)

As many as one million Americans suffer from CFS, although the cause of this mysterious illness is still unclear. What is becoming increasingly clearer is that for some CFS sufferers, alterations in the microbiome play a pivotal role, with many people being diagnosed after an infectious episode. Viral infections such as Epstein-Barr virus can damage the gut lining, creating a leaky gut mechanism that may explain the onset of CFS in some people. Low levels of *Bifidobacterium* coupled with higher-than-expected levels of oxygen-loving aerobic bacteria have been documented in CFS, suggesting a causative role for dysbiosis in at least some of these patients. Studies have also shown good responses to a typical dysbiosis/leaky gut dietary regimen, along with probiotic and glutamine supplementation, something I'll talk more about in Chapter 12.

Depression

Since gut microbes help digest food and assimilate nutrients, the question of which nutrients and other substances are available to the rest of your body depends on which species are present in your gut. Gut bacteria determine the availability of the precursor materials that your brain needs to make neurotransmitters, and they also communicate with a branch of the nervous system located in the GI tract called the enteric nervous system (ENS)—sometimes referred to as the second brain.

Gut bacteria are the main producers of serotonin, widely considered the body's feel-good hormone, which explains how our mental health is profoundly influenced by the health of our microbes. Mice who are separated from their mothers at birth exhibit depressive behavior and have lower-than-expected levels of *Lactobacillus* and *Bifidobacterium* species. Replacing these species increases their serotonin production and improves their markers of depression. Current therapies for depression in humans focus on manipulating serotonin levels, but boosting gut bacteria may be a more rational and successful approach. The link between gut bacteria and mood also explains why depression is an accompanying symptom to so many other forms of dysbiosis.

Skin Conditions

Microorganisms play a major role in noninfectious skin diseases such as acne, rosacea, and eczema. The ecosystem of bacteria, viruses, fungi, and mites that inhabit our skin and scalp consists of distinct microbial communities with different functions that for the most part live synergistically together. When we remove the protective bacteria as well as the natural oils and sebum that keep our skin supple and provide the ideal medium to nourish essential microbes, we create an unbalanced dysbiotic state on our skin. This allows pathogenic bacteria to overgrow, creating problems like cystic acne, rosacea, eczema, and dry, irritated skin, and increasing susceptibility to skin infections.

Antibacterial products that contain microbial disruptors like triclosan, over-washing with soap, too much shampooing, and the ubiquitous use of hand sanitizers can disrupt that ecosystem and lead to imbalances among the main bacterial species on our skin, as well as overgrowth of normally occurring populations such as the fungus *Malassezia*, which is associated with dandruff.

ACNE

Dermatologists routinely employ long courses of powerful antibiotics to treat acne, even though this condition is a classic example of dysbiosis of the skin: most doctors blame acne on the *Propionibacterium acnes* bacteria, but it's the overgrowth of *P. acnes* related to blockage of hair follicles and colonization with opportunistic bacteria such as *Staphylococcus aureus* that's the real problem, not the presence of *P. acnes* itself. Research shows that only *P. acnes* colonize healthy pores, while unhealthy ones universally include *Staphylococcus* and other bacterial undesirables. So it's really the alteration in the normal composition of skin microbes that leads to acne.

We're seeing more acne in young people these days—often as young as seven or eight years old, and many of them have a prior history of taking lots of antibiotics for ear infections or strep throat. Antibiotics are a temporary fix for acne that compounds the problem in the long run by leading to even more overgrowth of resistant species, which is why dermatologists often have to cycle acne patients through many different types of antibiotics as the bacteria grow more resistant.

Of all the different forms of dysbiosis I see, the patients who have been on years (sometimes decades!) of antibiotics for cystic acne are the most challenging to treat. Antibiotics such as erythromycin, doxycycline, minocycline, and tetracycline commonly used to treat acne have devastating effects on gut bacteria, and repopulating the colon can be an incredibly laborious effort. Their skin, like their gut, is ravaged by the onslaught of antibacterial agents, and they often develop superinfection on their face with yeast species as a result of the lack of essential bacteria. Antibiotic creams and lotions can be almost as damaging as antibiotics taken by mouth: *Clostridium difficile* (*C. diff*) is one of the side effects of Cleocin, a commonly prescribed topical antibiotic used for acne.

Studies show that more than half of all acne sufferers have significant alterations in gut flora, and societies that eat a microbiome-friendly diet with little or no processed foods or sugar have virtually no acne. While dermatologists are well meaning in their efforts to remediate what can be a devastating skin condition, especially in the teenage years, treating acne with antibiotics is one of our most damaging practices—something the medical community will likely look back on with real regret.

Hard to Undo

Glenn had been on various antibiotics for cystic acne for seventeen years. His skin would initially respond well, but after a year or two the cystic lesions would return, and his dermatologist would switch him to a different antibiotic. Ten years after he first started taking antibiotics Glenn began to have persistent loose stools and weight loss. He experimented with cutting out dairy and tried to increase his calories, but no matter what he ate, he still had diarrhea and trouble gaining weight. Evaluation of his digestive tract eventually revealed a diagnosis of celiac disease, and he was put on a GFD, which he adhered to strictly.

His doctor reassured Glenn that after a few months on the GFD his diarrhea and weight loss would improve, but two years later nothing had changed. Repeat evaluation showed the signs of celiac disease had completely resolved, and his small intestinal villi looked normal. But he didn't feel normal at all. In addition to the diarrhea and difficulty putting on weight, he had numbness in his lower extremities, headaches, brain fog, fatigue, and a host of other symptoms that no one seemed able to explain. He was prescribed antidepressant and antianxiety drugs, which didn't help and made him more tired. A shopping bag full of supplements prescribed by a local naturopath didn't help, either, and Glenn became more and more despondent about his health.

When Glenn came to see us, my nutritionist and I were particularly interested in what he was eating. The normal biopsies from his small intestine suggested that inadvertent gluten exposure wasn't the problem, but we wondered whether, like Mary in the earlier anecdote, he was eating a lot of nutrient-poor, gluten-free junk food. That wasn't the case, either. His diet incorporated lots of fruits and vegetables, some nuts and seeds, legumes, brown rice, quinoa, and a little lean animal protein, and really didn't leave much room for improvement. I checked his stool for evidence of yeast overgrowth and that was negative, too. I examined the rest of Glenn's digestive tract and found it all to be normal. Some microscopic forms of colitis can be associated with celiac disease, but he didn't have any of them. Every test we did came back negative, except the IP test for leaky gut, which was markedly positive, suggesting a significant increase in the permeability or "leakiness" of his gut membrane, something associated with both celiac disease and dysbiosis.

We put Glenn on a number of different diets, including ninety days of a strict anti-candida regimen that excludes most carbohydrates and is something I usually don't recommend. We dosed him up with our most robust prescription-strength probiotic. We tried glutamine supplements and oil of oregano (more on these in Chapter 12), and we pored over the results of his microbial stool analysis. In the end, it was clear that Glenn had severe dysbiosis, but we were unsuccessful in our efforts to reverse it. He had a little improvement with the interventions we recommended, but the majority of his symptoms were still present, and when last we heard from him he was contemplating entering a clinical trial of fecal transplantation for people with autoimmune diseases (more on this in Chapter 13).

Glenn had an extreme case of dysbiosis, no doubt brought on by almost two decades of antibiotic use that ultimately resulted in celiac disease as well as leaky gut. Most people with dysbiosis respond well to the regimen outlined in my Live Dirty, Eat Clean Plan, but there are times when microbial damage is simply too great to overcome. I remain optimistic that more novel and aggressive forms of microbiome rehab, like fecal transplantation, will ultimately prove successful in refractory cases like Glenn's.

ROSACEA

Rosacea is a form of autoimmune disease that's been linked to inflammation and bacterial imbalance in the gut. It's the most common skin condition in my bloated dysbiotic patients. In fact, one in twenty Americans suffers from it. Almost everyone I see with rosacea has a history of frequent antibiotic use or heavy topical therapy for acne, which can lead to damaged blood vessels that dilate easily, causing the flushed appearance typical of rosacea. Alcohol, sun exposure, extremes of temperature, spicy food, stress, and certain medications can trigger rosacea flare-ups, but many people also report a clear correlation between starchy, sugary food and their rosacea eruptions. Some studies suggest that bacteria-laden Demodex mites in the skin could be the cause of rosacea and have documented much higher levels of these mites on the skin of rosacea sufferers.

A topical antibiotic gel is the treatment of choice for rosacea in most dermatology offices, but eliminating processed grains and refined sugars from the diet seems to work even better for most of my patients, without the side effect of eventually making the condition worse by destroying essential bacteria.

ECZEMA

Eczema or atopic dermatitis (AD), the most common form, affects 15 percent of children in the United States and millions of adults. It's an immune-based problem that's frequently associated with other immune-related conditions, such as asthma and hay fever. After reading

Chapter 3, "The Hygiene Hypothesis and Our Modern Plagues," you're probably not surprised to hear that the incidence of eczema in industrialized countries has doubled over the past few decades.

Ninety percent of people with eczema are colonized with *Staphylococcus aureus*, compared to 5 percent of healthy people, and disease flares are often associated with a shift in skin microbes: a rise in the population of *Staphylococcus* species and a fall in overall microbial diversity. This dysbiotic skin state mirrors what we see in the gut with various diseases, including autoimmune conditions such as Crohn's and ulcerative colitis. Microbial diversity can decrease even further during flares of eczema, and studies have found that the less diversity present on the skin, the more severe the eczema. The standard treatment for eczema is steroids, which may temporarily suppress the inflammation, but ultimately exacerbate rather than address the root cause of the problem by contributing to the microbial imbalance.

Our skin is the first thing people notice when they see us, and when it's blemished or unhealthy-looking, it can significantly affect our self-esteem. But it's clear that neither dirt nor germs are the root cause of acne, rosacea, or eczema, and scrubbing away your essential skin microbes with harsh chemical potions, killing them off with antibiotics, or suppressing them with steroids isn't an effective or safe option. If you suffer from one of these skin conditions, consider taking a gentler, more holistic approach that nourishes rather than destroys your skin microbes and optimizes what you're feeding them through your own diet. My Live Dirty, Eat Clean Plan will show you how.

The Straw That Broke the Camel's Back: Lucia's Story

Lucia came to see me mainly to confirm that she was following the right path. She had had a healthy childhood but was treated with a year of tetracycline in high school for moderately severe acne. During the year she was on antibiotics she didn't feel quite right, with frequent nausea, an upset stomach, and cradle cap on the back of her scalp. Cradle cap, also known as seborrheic dermatitis, is a yellowish, crusty rash that's most common on the scalp of newborn babies, primarily as a result of yeast overgrowth. No one connected the cradle cap with Lucia's GI symptoms or suggested they might be related to the antibiotics.

In her twenties Lucia decided to see a gastroenterologist for her bouts of nausea, which had worsened after she started taking birth control pills. Biopsies taken during an upper endoscopy as part of the evaluation revealed the presence of *Helicobacter pylori* bacteria, a much-maligned inhabitant of the stomach. Under certain circumstances, *H. pylori* can be associated with ulcers or stomach cancer, but it's been a longtime resident of the stomach—around for millennia and present in half the world's population. We're just now realizing, thanks to the work of scientists such as Dr. Martin Blaser, that for many people, *H. pylori* has a protective effect, and its unnecessary eradication can lead to even more dangerous conditions such as esophageal inflammation and even cancer.

In Lucia's case, *Helicobacter pylori* was definitely not the cause of her nausea, and after two rounds of treatment, each lasting two weeks and consisting of three different antibiotics, her nausea was worse rather than better, and she started to develop reflux symptoms that she'd never had before—a known complication of *H. pylori* eradication in some people. That prompted her gastroenterologist to start her on acid suppression therapy, but not to question why a slim, otherwise healthy twenty-five-year-old who didn't smoke, drink, or eat big dinners late at night (which can create reflux problems) was suddenly having reflux. Lucia also developed recurrent episodes of the cradle cap she'd had in high school when taking the tetracycline for acne. Her doctor recommended a topical antifungal for the yeast problem, which would clear it up for a week or two before it came back again.

By this point Lucia was starting to lose faith in the medical community. Through her own self-study, she decided to stop the acid suppression, get off the birth control pills, and embark on a strict anti-candida diet that allowed only lean meats, fish, poultry, and green veg-

Dysbiosis—Do You Have It?   89

etables. The regimen was difficult to follow, and because she didn't have much of a taste for meat, she ate mostly vegetables. But by the end of the first week, she noticed a big difference in her symptoms. Her cradle cap was completely gone, her nausea was better, and the peculiar odor she'd noticed on her skin was also improved. After two weeks on the diet she liberalized what she was eating and continued to feel well, although she still avoided large amounts of sugary/starchy food, most fruits, and beans.

Two months after her recovery, Lucia developed a severe sore throat and low-grade fever. A swab for *Strep* came back positive. Reluctantly, she agreed to take antibiotics for a week. Within a few days of starting treatment, Lucia started to feel terrible again, with recurrence of all her previous symptoms. This time it took a month of strict dietary changes for her to get back to a good baseline. When I saw her in my office she was looking and feeling good, with no GI symptoms or manifestations of yeast overgrowth. I suggested that she liberalize her diet and reintroduce fruits and legumes. I also put her on a low dose of a probiotic to counter the microbiome-damaging effects of her recent course of antibiotics on top of the chronic antibiotic exposure she'd had as a teenager.

A five-day course of antibiotics can suppress as much as a third of your gut bacteria, and although many of the diminished species recover, not all do. For someone like Lucia, the excessive (and unnecessary) treatment for *H. pylori* was the straw that broke the camel's back, tipping her already altered microbiome into full-blown dysbiosis. Her ability to heal herself through changing her diet put her back in control of her health—the best place to be.

ALTHOUGH DYSBIOSIS DOESN'T cause everything that's wrong with us, I hope that after reading this chapter, you can see that it is at the heart of many of our common maladies, and the list of correlated conditions grows longer every day. Nurturing and caring for your microbes is a lot easier than trying to replace them when they're gone, but for those suffering from microbial discord, committing to dietary and lifestyle changes, understanding the role of probiotics (and sometimes even stool transplants), and learning how to avoid everyday microbial disruptors can mean light at the end of the tunnel. I'll explain how to accomplish it all in the Live Dirty, Eat Clean Plan.

Dysbiosis: Do You Have It?

Whether you've already been diagnosed with dysbiosis or one of its associated conditions, or are still trying to figure out the cause of your symptoms, this checklist will help you identify the root causes of what's gone wrong with your microbiome. Answering yes to even one of the questions from the list below could indicate you have dysbiosis, and the risk is cumulative based on how many risk factors you have.

TABLE 5–7 • Dysbiosis Checklist

Risk Factors for Dysbiosis:
- Have you taken **antibiotics** more than four times per year or for longer than two weeks at a time?
- Have you been on **birth control pills** or **hormone replacement therapy** in the last five years?
- Have you taken **corticosteroids** such as prednisone or cortisone for longer than two weeks at a time?
- Have you been on **acid suppressive therapy** with proton pump inhibitors or histamine blockers (H2 blockers) for more than a month at a time?
- Do you take **ibuprofen**, **aspirin**, or other **NSAIDs** regularly?
- When you were growing up, were you a **picky eater** who rarely ate green vegetables?
- Have you consumed large amounts of **sugar** and **starchy foods**?
- Do you drink more than ten **alcoholic beverages** per week?
- Do you drink one or more **sodas** or **diet sodas** daily?

- Have you ever had **diarrhea** or **dysentery** with **foreign travel**?
- Have you ever been diagnosed with a **parasite**?

Signs and Symptoms of Dysbiosis:

- Acne, eczema, rosacea
- Allergies and chronic food sensitivities
- Bad breath and gum disease
- Bloating or foul-smelling gas
- Brain fog
- Candida overgrowth or chronic yeast problems
- Chronic unexplained fatigue
- Depression or anxiety
- Difficulty losing weight
- Frequent colds, flu, or sinus infections
- Mucus in stool
- Poor digestion, including acid reflux
- Stomach bugs or episodes of food poisoning
- Unexplained diarrhea
- Vaginal or anal itching

Conditions Associated with Dysbiosis:

- Autoimmune disease
- Bacterial vaginosis (BV)
- Celiac disease or gluten sensitivity
- Diabetes
- Inflammatory bowel disease (IBD)
- Irritable bowel syndrome (IBS)
- Leaky gut
- Multiple sclerosis (MS)
- Obesity
- Small intestinal bacterial overgrowth (SIBO)
- Sinusitis
- Thyroid disease
- Yeast infections

CHAPTER 6

||||||||||||||||||||||||||||||||||||||||||

Are Our Bacteria Making Us Fat?

O BESITY HAS INCREASED dramatically in the past few decades: more than one-third of adults in the United States and almost one in five children are obese, and fully one-third of the population worldwide is overweight. The rates have increased too rapidly for us to blame our weight problem on our genes, and although a diet high in fat and sugar is partly responsible, even that doesn't account for the striking increase in body mass index. Maintaining a stable weight seems to be much more complicated than calories in versus calories out. It's what happens to those calories as they pass through our thirty-foot digestive superhighway that may explain why so many of us are gaining weight.

Gut Bacteria Determine Weight

We can distinguish between leanness and obesity with 90 percent accuracy just from looking at gut bacteria. Obese mice have a higher ratio of *Firmicutes* to *Bacteroidetes* phyla compared to their lean counterparts, as well as reduced microbial diversity, and the same seems to be true of obese humans. Several experiments have shown that when we transplant microbes from obese mice into germ-free lean mice, they gain weight and their fat deposition increases, without any change in their diet or exercise regimen.

As I explained in Chapter 5, microbes from obese mice—and from people, too—seem to be able to extract more calories from the same food. Although we're not sure exactly how this happens, there are a number of ways bacteria can change their energy harvest: by controlling the transit time of food through the digestive tract, which determines how many calories can be extracted and absorbed; by influencing hormones that determine whether calories are deposited as fat versus used as energy; and by themselves consuming extra calories for tissue repair or other tasks. And it's not just energy that's extracted differently; certain microbiomes are able to extract more nutrients from food, too, which can be advantageous in situations where nutrient-dense foods are scarce. People colonized with gut bacteria that are more efficient at breaking down food are able to absorb more calories and end up gaining more weight, while bacteria that are not as good at extracting calories are associated with leanness.

Although we don't yet know exactly what a "lean microbiome" looks like, we're learning more about which species are associated with leanness and which diets may cultivate those species. Researchers have identified a family of bacteria called *Christensenellaceae* that seem to help people stay lean. Mice transplanted with these microbes tend to gain less weight than untreated mice eating the same diet. *Christensenellaceae* are only one example of probably hundreds of different microbes—some previously described and others not yet discovered— whose presence may impact our weight.

Gut bacteria can also lead to malnutrition. A study in Malawi looked at the gut bacteria in sets of identical twins where one was well nourished and the other malnourished. It turned out that these genetically identical individuals had different microbiomes: the malnourished children couldn't synthesize certain vitamins or digest complex carbohydrates properly. Transplanting microbes from the malnourished twins into germ-free mice created the same deficiencies, confirming that bacteria can cause malnutrition, even in the presence of an adequate diet. Therefore, just as some microbes can extract more calories and nutrients from the same food, some microbes can extract less.

Dysbiosis Can Make You Fat

We all know people who eat a lot of food, rarely exercise, and hardly gain a pound, and others who restrict calories, work out all the time, and still struggle with their weight. In my practice, many of the people I see with dysbiosis are in the latter category. Yeast overgrowth can cause excessive and hard-to-control cravings for sugary, starchy foods, which can lead to weight gain. But even after eliminating those foods, following an extremely restricted diet, and getting plenty of exercise, many people continue to have a difficult time losing weight because they're still colonized with the wrong bacteria. Restoring a healthy mix of microbes can be an essential part of getting their weight under control.

Studies in overweight children show a reduction in beneficial bacteria such as *Bifidobacteria* and an increase in pathogens like *Staphylococcus aureus* and *Enterobacteriaceae*. The bacterial composition of the gut in overweight adolescents can influence how much weight they lose with dietary restriction and increased physical activity independent of their diet, confirming that the microbiome is an incredibly important factor in determining the efficacy of dietary interventions.

What About Your Genes?

Your genes definitely have some influence on how easily you gain or lose weight, especially on where you gain it, helping dictate whether you end up a belly-prominent apple or a thigh-heavy pear. But your microbes may actually have more say than your genes in whether you end up overweight or not.

Researchers at Washington University in St. Louis took gut bacteria from identical twins, where one was lean and one was obese, and transplanted them into germ-free mice. Within weeks, the mice that received microbes from the obese twin became obese, and the ones that received microbes from the lean twin stayed lean, validating the concept that our microbes, not our genes, may be primarily responsible for changes in our weight.

Does Food Make a Difference?

The food you eat clearly affects the composition of the bacterial communities in your gut—high-fat, low-fiber diets are associated with a very different microbial profile than low-fat, high-fiber diets—and that microbial composition can in turn influence whether or not you end up gaining weight. Since bacteria follow the food, instead of counting calories when we're trying to slim down, a model that clearly falls short in accounting for weight gain or loss, we should be looking at how to shape our microbiome in a way that influences caloric extraction from food.

Cutting down on processed grains and refined sugar can affect our microbiome in a positive way, but replacing those foods with too much animal protein and fat can be problematic, because they may crowd out the dietary fibers that are an important component of a microbiome associated with leanness. I see a plateau in weight loss in many of my patients who put themselves on restrictive low-carb diets or Paleo devotees who don't eat enough vegetables, probably because they're not cultivating the right microbes. I'll go into more detail about the ideal mix of nutrients needed to optimize your microbiome and maintain a healthy weight in Chapter 9.

Is Our Super-sanitized Lifestyle Making Us Fat?

It may seem hard to believe, but obesity is one of the consequences of our super-sanitized lifestyle.

H. PYLORI

Less than 10 percent of school-age children now harbor *Helicobacter pylori*, a number that's decreased dramatically from decades ago as a result of widespread use of antibiotics. In later life, *H. pylori* may be associated with stomach ulcers and other problems, but in childhood it seems to have a more protective effect, including keeping ghrelin in check; ghrelin is the "hunger hormone" produced in the gastrointestinal (GI) tract that makes us want to eat. Without *H. pylori*'s influence on ghrelin, children may be missing the cues that tell them when to stop eating.

ANTIBIOTICS

Studies show that children prescribed large amounts of antibiotics are at higher risk for obesity later in life. Antibiotic exposure before birth can be a major hazard, too: antibiotic use in pregnant women in the second and third trimesters is associated with an increased risk of obesity in their babies. In animal studies, combining antibiotics with a high-fat diet seems to be a synergistic factor that's associated with even more rapid weight gain, and the same is true in humans.

CHEMICALS

Triclosan is an antimicrobial agent found in consumer products such as soaps, detergents, and some brands of toothpaste. Despite being marketed as antibacterial, household soaps and sanitizers containing triclosan don't offer any real benefit over conventional soap and water, but they may confer additional risk, including higher rates of food allergies and a higher body mass index.

You Can't Hack Your Microbiome

While it may seem that a simple solution to the obesity epidemic (and lots of our other problems) is to just replace our not-so-great microbes with better ones, it turns out that's not so easily done. Gut bacteria have a very short life span—just minutes, in many cases. Even though we can temporarily change our microbial composition by inoculating ourselves with different bugs, we tend to revert to our "old" microbiome pretty quickly, so creating lasting change can be a challenging process.

Even if we swap out our microbes for ones associated with leanness, if we're not eating the right mix of foods to nourish and sustain those microbes, they're not going to survive or reproduce for very long. In the Live Dirty, Eat Clean Plan, I'll give you specific recommendations and recipes to help you incorporate more microbe-boosting foods into your diet—an essential step in maintaining a natural, healthy weight.

CHAPTER 7

||||||||||||||||||||||||||||||||||||||||

Modern Microbial Disruptors

SOME SCIENTISTS ARGUE that the dramatic differences in our microbiome today simply represent evolutionary adaptations to our changing environment. They maintain that there is no ideal microbiome, just the one that's evolved with us. But as I've discussed throughout this book, much of what's happening to our microbes isn't just benign manifestations of our changing environment; they're also extremely detrimental to our health and are often a result of modern practices that are incorrectly promoted as being beneficial and necessary when profit and convenience are the real motivators, or of scientific innovations that haven't been sufficiently assessed through rigorous testing to exclude the possibility of harm to microbial health—a concept still in its infancy.

Medical Practices and Modern Mind-sets

Medical procedures that were designed for emergency situations are now routinely employed, and it's commonplace to treat healthy people with antibiotics to prevent infection that would likely occur in only a few. Let's take a closer look at some of the more common medical practices that disrupt our microbial well-being.

Cesarean Sections

Julius Caesar was allegedly cut from his ailing mother's womb, and legend has it that a subsequent Roman decree allowed C-sections to be used to save infants when the mother was dead or dying. The notion that a woman could survive this type of surgery didn't take hold until the late 1800s, but even then, C-sections were performed only in dire circumstances with very low expectations of the mother surviving.

The rate of C-sections in the United States is now one in three births. While some are medically necessary for reasons such as fetal distress, breech position, umbilical cord prolapse, and uterine rupture, a growing number are based on convenience, commerce, and the widespread use of labor-inducing drugs (which speed up the final hours of a process that takes nine months from start to finish, evolved over millions of years, results in the production of a brand-new human being, and arguably should not be rushed). Maternal outcomes have improved a lot in the last century, but C-sections still come with plenty of risk, particularly to our fragile blossoming microbiome.

As I mentioned in Chapter 1, babies born vaginally are colonized with *Lactobacillus* species and other essential microbes from their mother as they pass through the birth canal. C-section babies miss out on this important step and are typically colonized with less desirable hospital bacteria. Lower levels of these protective microbes mean that babies born via C-section have higher rates of asthma, allergies, type 1 diabetes, and other autoimmune conditions. Studies also show an almost 50 percent increase in risk for obesity in C-section babies. Being born via C-section and receiving antibiotics early in life, which happens to many children these days, is a double whammy associated with an even higher risk for being obese—and sick—later on.

My daughter genuinely wanted to know if she could be rebirthed, since she was a C-section baby the first time around. But the timing of the colonization is key. It can't be redone with the same results as an adult or even a mature child.

Although we don't get a second chance to make our first appearance, microbiologist Maria Gloria Dominguez-Bello, PhD, and others have come up with a way to give C-section babies a shot at those microbes they're missing out on. It's a simple but brilliant idea: wipe down C-section babies immediately after delivery with gauze that's been doused in their mother's vaginal juices, in order to colonize them with essential bacteria from their mother's birth canal. In our modern medical industrial complex, we do the exact opposite of what nature intended—we obsessively clean our babies right after birth, wiping away the newly minted microbes that are their main source of protection.

Medical innovations such as C-sections can be lifesaving, but the risk-benefit analysis changes dramatically when they're used indiscriminately. Our medical training encourages us to be early adopters of practices perceived as beneficial, which often occurs before the evidence accrues. The convenience of a scheduled C-section can't be denied: you can pick the person you want to do the delivery, the place, and the time, while avoiding the unpredictability of a vaginal birth. But besides the hit to the baby's microbiome, C-sections come with lots of risks to the mother, too: infection, bleeding, blood clots, injury to the bladder or bowel, higher rates of complications in future pregnancies, and a death rate triple that of vaginal deliveries. As for the baby, being yanked out before nature intended can increase the chances of breathing problems and a stay in the neonatal intensive care unit.

Giving birth is one of our most innate and natural abilities, but having a baby has become a highly medicalized experience, even for those at very low risk for complications. The pros and cons of C-sections are really worth thinking about if you're planning to have children or are pregnant and considering how you'd like to give birth. Having a plan for your baby's delivery that lays out precisely what you'd like to happen (barring any unexpected complications) is a great idea, given the consequences of unnecessary medical intervention. I'll give you some tips on how to accomplish this in the Live Dirty, Eat Clean Plan, including a birth plan that you can customize to fit your needs.

Antibiotics in Pregnancy

Almost half of all women giving birth in U.S. hospitals and almost all of those undergoing C-section receive antibiotics. Most are treated because of colonization with group B strep (GBS) or other potential, not actual, infections. GBS is present in the vaginas of about 25 percent of healthy women, so lots of pregnant women test positive for it. The overwhelming majority of babies born to GBS-positive mothers are completely healthy, but in about one in two hundred births, GBS may be associated with serious illness. So, to prevent potential problems in a small percentage of babies, we prophylactically (i.e., preventively) treat large numbers of healthy, asymptomatic women with antibiotics during late pregnancy or delivery, exposing them and their newborn babies to these drugs.

Most are never specifically asked whether they'd like to be treated, or told that they have been (the consent you sign when you're admitted to the hospital usually includes general statements about need for medications, not specifics about each drug administered). And they're certainly not typically informed about the hazards of exposing their newborn to broad-spectrum antibiotics that kill everything in their path, including their baby's newly acquired and essential microbes.

If antibiotics were benign, treating many to prevent illness in a few wouldn't be such a bad idea, but that's definitely not the case. As discussed in Chapter 4, "Pharmageddon and the Antibiotic Paradox," the undeniable fact is that antibiotics kill both bad and good microbes indiscriminately—GBS as well as the vital *Lactobacillus* population—paradoxically rendering those who are treated *more* rather than less prone to subsequent infection because of the reduction in protective species. Babies exposed to antibiotics as newborns have an 84 percent increase in risk for obesity because of the effect on their developing microbiome and, like C-section babies, much higher rates of asthma, allergies, and autoimmune diseases later in life. If you're contemplating conception, it's important to keep in mind that if you're exposed to antibiotics during pregnancy, not only will your microflora be abnormal, but your baby's will be, too.

Baby Formula

The fact that women are able to produce food for their babies and carry it around with them inside their body with no need for refrigeration, bottles, or sterilizers is an incredible design feat. What's even more incredible is the synergy between breast milk and the baby's microbiome. Indigestible carbohydrates in breast milk feed the baby's essential microbes, which in turn repel unfriendly bacteria on the mother's nipple.

Breast-feeding is a crucial part of our development as humans and as microbial hosts, and we see big differences when it's skipped in favor of formula. Formula-fed babies who don't get any breast milk have a 20 percent lower survival rate than breast-fed babies, and in countries with poor sanitation, the difference is even greater. Like babies born by C-section, formula-fed babies also have higher rates of allergy, asthma, and autoimmune diseases. Given these statistics, encouraging formula over breast milk in developing countries that already have high rates of infant mortality is particularly egregious.

There are undoubtedly countless additional undiscovered ingredients in breast milk that are designed to nourish the baby's microbiome, which is why artificially made formula really can't compare and why we continue to see the health benefits of nursing long after babies are weaned and well into adulthood.

Some health care practitioners present breast-feeding as a personal choice, telling women it's perfectly fine if they prefer not to breast-feed and suggesting that formula is an equivalent option. For those who are unable to nurse for medical reasons or who don't have adequate breast milk, supplementing with formula is certainly a reasonable option, but given what we know about the benefits, there should be whole clinics devoted to teaching women how to breast-feed and making sure they understand the importance of nursing or expressing as much breast milk as possible for their babies—and the potential consequences of not doing so.

Modern Mind-sets

Like many people, I thought of nonemergency C-sections, baby formula, and preventive antibiotics as modern medical advances that at the very least cause no harm and are probably beneficial. I learned the hard way that nothing could be further from the truth.

Mine was an uneventful and healthy pregnancy, but I had the flu and a low-grade fever when I went into labor, so the doctors gave me antibiotics "just in case" there was something else going on that actually needed treating. I'd never been a hospital patient before, so being on the receiving end of things was a new experience. Lying flat on my back with an intrauterine monitor threaded up through my vagina, an additional external fetal heart rate monitor strapped to my belly, drugs to make my uterus contract harder coursing through my veins, and a catheter dripping anesthetic into my spine, I realized that having a baby nowadays was a far cry from what nature intended. I was glad that all this monitoring and medication was available, but I did have a sense that there was something incongruous about these measures being employed in a healthy person.

After fourteen hours of labor, I was told it was time for a C-section, something I wanted to avoid mostly because the post-op recovery time would interfere with my running, and avoiding surgery if you didn't need it seemed like a good idea (the microbial disadvantages weren't yet on my radar!). Despite my best efforts to persuade the medical team otherwise, I was told there was no other choice but to proceed with the C-section.

After the C-section, the pediatrician did a thorough assessment and found my daughter, Sydney, to be in good health, but because of my flu and low-grade fever, she was whisked off to the neonatal intensive care unit (NICU) for observation. It turned out that "observation" included a spinal tap, blood cultures, analysis of her urine, and administration of two potent intravenous antibiotics.

At the time, I was thrilled that the doctors were being so proactive and giving her antibiotics "just in case." I still wholeheartedly believed in the wonders of modern medicine and, like most doctors a decade ago, I was unaware of the long-term risks of antibiotics. What happened next was a series of events that I now realize were clearly related to my C-section and the antibiotics that Sydney and I received, and I wish I had a reset button to do it all over differently.

I nursed Sydney for the first six weeks after she was born. Then my breast milk dried up and we had to switch to formula. She didn't tolerate the initial product (high-fructose genetically modified corn solids were the main ingredient), so our pediatrician advised that we switch to soy. Had I known at the time that a day's worth of soy formula contained the estrogen equivalent of a few birth control pills, I'm pretty sure I would have vetoed that recommendation, but I was a dutiful patient following what I thought was sage advice from my doctor.

A few months after birth, Sydney had her first of what would be many, many upper respiratory tract and ear infections. Each time, she was prescribed stronger and stronger antibiotics for longer periods of time. By the time she was three, she had received more than a dozen courses of antibiotics, and after a visit for a lingering cough led to a diagnosis of asthma and more prescriptions—this time steroids, an antihistamine, a bronchodilator, and an antibiotic—I decided it was time for another approach.

I'm an advocate of not fixing it if it ain't broke, but in this case it was broke from too much fixing. We decided to stop the cycle of doctor visits and antibiotics and give Sydney's little body a chance to recover. And recover she did, although it took a few years, lots of green smoothies, and big dietary changes. She still gets high fevers and takes a long time to recover when she has a virus, but overall, she's a healthy ten-year-old who hasn't taken an antibiotic in several years.

I recognize that hospitals and medical professionals help countless sick people every day, but my greatest regret is that, as a healthy person, I got tangled up in the medical industrial complex and allowed my child to be exposed to all those unnecessary and harmful antibiotics. Knowing what I now know about the conditions associated with C-section delivery, formula, and being given lots of antibiotics at a young age, I still worry that Sydney will develop an autoimmune disease such as Crohn's or have manifestations of leaky gut as she gets older.

My reset button if I had the chance to do it all over would be a vaginal delivery at home with a well-trained midwife, at least a year of breast milk before transitioning to homemade plant-based baby food, and no antibiotics unless she had a life-threatening infection. I'm not suggesting this should be the standard for every woman—lots of people benefit from closer monitoring in a hospital setting, judicious use of pain medication and other drugs during labor, and having lots of trained professionals around. But it is important for those of us giving birth to know that less medical intervention is an option and often the safer choice in the long run. My customizable birth plan in Chapter 11 offers helpful information on how to achieve a more holistic childbirth.

Fortunately, the microbiome is ever changing, and although Sydney started out microbially disadvantaged, I suspect we've made up a lot of the difference through careful attention to diet and lifestyle. "Live dirty, eat clean" is the mantra in our household, and so far it seems to be working.

Appendectomy

For decades, medical practitioners have considered the appendix an unnecessary vestigial organ with no real purpose other than getting inflamed and requiring surgical removal. But it turns out that the appendix plays a very important role: it's where extra good bacteria get stored for when we really need them, like after an episode of traveler's diarrhea or a viral illness. Think of it as a microbial reservoir of sorts that can help to repopulate the gastrointestinal (GI) tract.

Surgeons often have a low threshold for an appendectomy, sometimes making the decision to remove it during abdominal exploration even in the absence of obvious inflammation. We've seen other examples in medicine where this sort of "just in case" mentality led to poor outcomes—women who were plunged into premature menopause after their reproductive organs were removed because they'd finished having children and their uterus was therefore considered no longer necessary. Just as the uterus has other functions besides making babies (it directs blood flow to the pelvis and genitalia during sexual intercourse), so, too, the appendix is turning out to be an important player in our microbial health and well-being.

Everyday Microbial Disruptors

Some of the most problematic practices are the ones we employ every day in our endless quest for cleanliness. A major part of rehabbing our microbiome and restoring our health is recognizing that cleaner doesn't mean better; in fact, it can sometimes mean worse.

Hand Sanitizers

Although the number of species in and on our bodies increases as we age, our diversity of species is highest during childhood. Being colonized with lots of different microbes is actually good for us, and scrubbing them away with the chemicals in most hand sanitizers does us far more harm than good. Products marketed as "antibacterial" have absolutely no advantage over regular soap and water—and it's a good idea to use soap and water if you're around people who are sick or in a hospital setting. Like the overuse of antibiotics, our obsession with sanitizers is a particularly bad idea, knocking out important species that sometimes never fully recover, and leading to a less diverse, frailer microbiome.

I marvel at the amount of hand sanitizer used in most schools today and try to convince fellow parents that they're much better off allowing their children to eat a little dirt from the playground than to ingest triclosan and other chemicals from their sanitized hands. Kids are supposed to get dirty—it's how we know they're running around outside playing, getting exercise, and having a good time. I worry if my daughter arrives home from school too clean; it makes me wonder what she's been doing all day. Most children's natural inclination to play in the dirt and their complete lack of concern for cleanliness are things we should be cherishing and encouraging—I believe these traits are part of our innate Darwinian survival code to help build and maintain a healthy microbiome. I'll share some advice on how to rewild your child—and yourself—in the Live Dirty, Eat Clean Plan.

Chlorinated Drinking Water

Routine chlorination of public drinking water began in the early 1900s as a way to prevent outbreaks of cholera and typhoid fever, and although widespread chlorination has been successful at reducing the spread of waterborne diseases, it's come at a cost to our beneficial bacteria, as even low levels of chlorine are very toxic to essential microbes.

Water filters designed for home use can remove most of the chlorine in tap water, as well as parasites such as giardia that may contaminate older water filtration systems and can survive low levels of chlorination. But treated water that's been filtered still takes a toll on our microbiome, and in addition to chlorine, it can contain hundreds of different pollutants—including antibiotics. Perhaps a better idea would be to test for harmful pathogens, such as cholera and typhoid, and put probiotics in the water supply instead of antibiotics and chemicals such as chlorine, in an effort to repopulate rather than deplete our already dwindling microbes.

Agricultural Practices

We've reached the tragic era where our children are expected to live shorter lives than we did, despite all of our medical advances and technology. The decrease in life expectancy parallels the shift from family to factory farming, and dramatic changes in how we produce what we eat. Most people born in the first half of the twentieth century ate food grown within a few miles of where they lived—if not in their own backyard. Lacing the food with microbial disruptors, such as antibiotics, hormones, and pesticides, or genetically modifying the food itself wasn't yet common practice.

Animals, Antibiotics, and Growth Promotion

Antibiotics have been routinely given to some animals raised for human consumption since the 1950s as a way to promote growth. A whopping 80 percent of all antibiotics sold in the United States are used in the livestock and poultry industry, either to enhance growth in healthy animals or to prevent infection because the animals are being raised in crowded, unsanitary conditions that increase the risk of illness. Altering gut bacteria, as happens with ingestion of antibiotics, can increase weight by as much as 15 percent in farm animals—and the same is likely true for the people who eat them. As we discussed in the last chapter, overweight and normal-sized people have significantly different microbiomes, and antibiotics can induce many of those differences.

Using antibiotics preventively in confined animals leads to drug-resistant bacteria that pose a real threat to human health. Because genes that confer resistance can be passed from bacteria in farm animals to bacteria in our digestive tracts, many of the drugs in our antibiotic arsenal that we really need for treating infection in humans end up being ineffective. We've seen outbreaks of resistant *E. coli* and methicillin-resistant *Staphylococcus aureus* (MRSA) that can be traced back to the livestock industry, although overuse of antibiotics in hospitals also contributes to the problem of drug resistance. There's very little transparency from the Food and Drug Administration (FDA), pharmaceutical manufacturers, or animal breeders when it comes to disclosing which antibiotics are being used, and for which indications, but the fact that every year inspections of meat and poultry reveal more resistance to antibiotics is a dire warning of what the future may look like.

PESTICIDES

Most pesticides used in the food industry aren't well absorbed in humans, so they may not pose a direct risk to us, but some studies suggest that chemicals such as glyphosate can disrupt metabolic pathways in our microbes. Some of the more pathogenic bacteria like *Clostridium* and *Salmonella* seem to be resistant to glyphosate, while essential bacteria like *Lactobacillus* and *Bifidobacterium* are often more susceptible, which can lead to an unbalanced microbiome and dysbiosis (see Chapter 5).

Genetic Modification

Bacillus thuringiensis (Bt) is a bacterium that lives in soil and produces a toxin that kills insects by making their intestines burst. Biotech companies have inserted the gene for Bt toxin into foods such as corn so that the crop can produce its own insecticide. It's an example of genetic modification: the process of taking genetic material from one organism and inserting it into the permanent genetic code of another. Bt corn has found its way into most processed food and drinks through the widespread use of high fructose corn syrup. It's also in most commercially produced livestock that's been fed Bt corn on factory farms.

In an ideal world, Bt toxin would kill insects but get destroyed in our digestive tracts. But a Canadian study found that Bt toxin was present in 93 percent of pregnant women tested, 80 percent of umbilical blood in their babies, and 67 percent of nonpregnant women. Other studies have confirmed that genes inserted into genetically modified food such as Bt corn can be transferred to our gut bacteria by a process known as conjugation. So instead of being destroyed, the Bt toxin may actually be present in our bodies, and, through gene transfer, bacteria in our digestive tract may be able to synthesize it.

Scientists have found a wide range of immune responses in mice fed Bt corn, including elevated antibodies, and white blood cells of the kind typically associated with allergic and autoimmune reactions. This has led researchers to wonder whether the dramatic increase we're seeing in allergic and inflammatory conditions could be related to some of these genetically modified substances.

I wonder about the same thing in many of my patients with irritable bowel syndrome, food allergies, leaky gut, and dysbiosis. Their symptoms frequently seem to be correlated with something they're eating, but we just can't put our finger on what it is, and many of them describe feeling "poisoned." Spray insecticides can be washed off food, but genetically inserted toxins such as Bt, in addition to being modified from their naturally occurring state, are part of the food we eat—they can't be separated or avoided.

In 2010 the American Academy of Environmental Medicine recommended that physicians tell their patients to exclude genetically modified foods from their diets. Like many other organizations, they also called for more independent long-term safety studies and labeling of foods that contain genetically modified ingredients. We're still learning about the long-term effects of genetic modification of our food. My approach for patients with dysbiosis is to recommend excluding these foods from their diet, not because there is a clear link, but because there might be.

Seeing Our World with New Eyes

I'm not advocating that we abandon modern medicine or agricultural techniques that improve the efficiency of food production. But I am suggesting that we pay careful attention to the effect these practices have not just on our own health but on the health of our microbial roommates. When most of these practices were first adopted, nobody really knew anything about the microbiome or how intricately tied it was to our own health. Now that we do, we have a real obligation to evaluate things differently—to consider not just the economic advantages of modern practices, or their convenience, or the fact that they make our lives more comfortable. We have to ask ourselves whether how we're living helps or hinders our microbes, because that's what ultimately informs our own health.

part 3

REWILDING
OURSELVES

CHAPTER 8

||||||||||||||||||||||||||||||||||||||||

Introducing the
Live Dirty, Eat Clean Plan

I N THE LAST century alone, we've destroyed more than 80 percent of the earth's forests, fully exploited or depleted 70 percent of the world's fish, and lost half of the wild animals on the planet. We're in the midst of the worst species die-off since the dinosaurs disappeared, losing animals at a rate thousands of times faster than what should naturally be occurring. The loss of species and their natural habitats leads to an imbalanced ecosystem in which drought, famine, and global warming become part of the normal landscape. Species further down on the food chain grow out of control when their natural predators are diminished, and huge ecological gaps develop when unsound environmental practices become a way of life.

In conservation biology, "rewilding" means the reintroduction of species into areas where they've become extinct, with the goal of returning to a more natural and balanced existence. It's an important part of repairing and restoring our relationship with the natural world—not just the one we live in but also the one that lives inside us. Just as conservation efforts of reforestation, protecting wildlife, and replenishing the oceans are essential to life on the planet, so re-creating a balanced microbial habitat in our bodies might be the single most important step in improving our individual and collective health.

But how exactly do we rewild ourselves? What do we need to do to restore and maintain a densely populated, healthy microbiome, with the right mix of species all working together? Is it possible to provide nourishing food for our gut bacteria without having to grow it all ourselves? Can infections be treated or prevented without antibiotics? What about modern practices that make our lives convenient and comfortable but wipe out legions of essential bacteria in the process? Is it possible to get back to a dirtier, healthier way of life, while still living in the modern world?

Remove, Replace, Restore

The cornerstone of the Live Dirty, Eat Clean Plan is *removing* medications, practices, and foods that are damaging to your microbiome; *replacing* the essential bacteria that you've lost with a robust probiotic; and *restoring* the health of your gut with appropriate nutrients, supplements, and medicinal foods.

The good news is you don't have to go all the way back to the cave to rewild yourself, although my Live Dirty, Eat Clean Plan will show you how to bring some important elements of cave life back home. If you suffer from any of the manifestations of dysbiosis I've discussed, have been diagnosed with an autoimmune disease, struggle with your weight, or want to safeguard against future illness, this plan will provide you with everything you need to achieve optimal microbial health: what to eat, lifestyle tactics, how to approach illness, a guide to probiotics and supplements, and important details about fecal transplants—the next frontier in medicine. Here's a preview of what you can expect on the Plan:

- Chapter 9, "The Live Dirty, Eat Clean Diet," introduces a whole new way of looking at food that emphasizes the nutrients you need to grow a good gut garden. It combines the best of how our Paleolithic ancestors ate with microbe-boosting, plant-based strategies, and it has helped thousands of my patients with dysbiosis recover and heal. The food is simple to prepare because it's enjoyed in its natural state. The plan is easy to adhere to because there's no calorie counting, and the focus is on what you're missing and need to add in rather than on what you should eliminate. Using food as the nourishing medicine that it's meant to be will optimize your microbiome, help you achieve and maintain your ideal weight, boost your energy levels, and improve your overall health, all while enjoying easy-to-assemble, delicious meals.

- Chapter 10, "The Live Dirty Lifestyle," gives you practical rewilding advice for everyday life, from simple things like throwing out the hand sanitizer and opening a window, to specific details like which ingredients to avoid in personal care products. You'll learn how to groom and care for yourself without stripping away the microbial soil that's the key to cultivating healthy hair and skin, and become familiar with microbiome-friendly recipes for beauty products straight from the garden and kitchen. I'll share the Live Dirty dos and don'ts that I follow in my own life that can help rewild you, your family, and your home.

- Chapter 11, "A Rewilding Approach to Illness," provides you with strategies for tackling health challenges without destroying precious microbes in the process. It includes a list of the critical questions to ask your doctor when you're sick, advice on how to protect your microbes when you're taking an antibiotic, a primer on which medications are detrimental to essential bacteria and should be avoided, and microbe-sparing remedies for common ailments such as acne, urinary tract infections, and chronic sinus problems. I'll also outline a birth plan for expectant mothers to help avoid the pitfalls of antibiotics during pregnancy, unnecessary C-sections, the use of baby formula, and other practices that damage your baby's burgeoning microbiome.

- Chapter 12, "Bugs over Drugs: Probiotics and Other Supplements," explains exactly what to look for in a probiotic—how much live bacteria should be present, which species and strains are the most beneficial, and how long you need to take it. I'll also explain which nutritional supplements can help restore and replenish your microbiome and share options for obtaining those ingredients naturally from food and herbs.

- Chapter 13, "Everything You Wanted to Know About Stool Transplants but Were Afraid to Ask," explains FMT—fecal microbiota transplant—including the pros and cons, appropriate indications, ideal donor profile, testing required, and how to actually perform a fecal transplant at home (hint: get a friend to help!). Most people will never need to be on the receiving end of a fecal transplant, but once you get beyond the yuck factor and understand the science behind FMT, you'll realize why this procedure is becoming such an important medical resource for people with severe forms of dysbiosis.

CHAPTER 9

||||||||||||||||||||||||||||||||||||||||||

The Live Dirty,
Eat Clean Diet

All Disease Begins in the Gut

Hippocrates said it thousands of years before I did, and he was right. Much, if not all, disease begins in the gut, and that's especially true for the modern diseases that plague us today. That's why in integrative or holistic medicine, the protocols for treating different conditions are often so similar. Whether you're dealing with Crohn's, psoriasis, multiple sclerosis (MS), rheumatoid arthritis, leaky gut, or eczema, chances are you've come across compelling evidence suggesting that eliminating refined sugar, processed grains like gluten, genetically modified corn products, and dairy can help improve your condition. Some practitioners refer to this approach as *healing from the inside* or *identifying the root cause of disease.* More and more, that root cause looks like a distressed microbiome, and one of the most successful and least toxic ways to heal it is to alter what's going on in your gut by drastically changing the way you've been eating. It works for dysbiosis and for related conditions where an altered microbiome plays a key role.

Food as Medicine, and Lessons from Lydia

In the early days of my career as a gastroenterologist, I looked askance when patients told me they were treating their Crohn's disease or ulcerative colitis by changing their diet. Not taking medication when you had a serious illness struck me as irresponsible and risky, like driving without car insurance—what if you got into an accident? I'd do my best to convince people, even those who were feeling well, that they still needed drugs, just in case. But ultimately I was the one who was convinced otherwise.

Back then, many patients were wary (and some still are) about telling their doctors if they were self-treating with dietary changes, supplements, or mind-body techniques. They worried about being perceived as noncompliant or uncooperative. In 2000, when I was a full-time faculty member at Georgetown Hospital, I administered an anonymous questionnaire to patients in my IBD (inflammatory bowel disease) clinic to evaluate the use of complementary and alternative practices. I found that 70 percent of patients were using one or more practices, often in conjunction with prescription medication, but usually on a "don't ask, don't tell" basis. Well, I decided I would ask. I started asking patients "what else" they were doing to feel better. I was amazed at how many people were getting additional relief from changing how they ate, having regular acupuncture treatments, and getting into the habit of doing meditation.

My first patient whose aggressive Crohn's disease went into remission using diet alone left an indelible impression and set me on a path to find out how far nutritional therapy could take me and my patients. Lydia was a nurse at Georgetown, and in addition to my being her doctor, we were about the same age and good friends. I'd diagnosed her with aggressive Crohn's disease involving both the colon and small intestine, and although we'd initiated therapy with a benign anti-inflammatory drug, her disease had progressed quickly, requiring more potent medications. We finally got her symptoms under control using a monoclonal antibody drug—a therapy that's often effective but comes with the price tag of an increased risk of serious infections and lymphoma—but she still had occasional episodes of diarrhea and abdominal pain.

Lydia moved away for two years to take a job at another hospital, and when she came back, her Crohn's symptoms were completely gone. She looked happy and healthy and full of energy. I was amazed but skeptical when she told me she was on no medications and was eating primarily vegetables, fruit, nuts, a little bit of lean animal protein, lentils, and the occasional bowl of rice. I was delighted that she was feeling well, but I kept waiting for her to have a flare-up or to find signs of active disease on her colonoscopy. It never happened. Lydia remained on her diet; aside from some scarring, her colon looked normal each time I examined it; and her disease remained in remission.

Lydia was the first of many IBD patients I had the privilege of caring for whose disease was controlled by changing their diet, and she opened my eyes to what was possible. I wasn't just skeptical but downright afraid in the beginning. I felt a moral obligation as a physician to convince my patients that whatever dietary changes they made needed to be undertaken in conjunction with drug therapy, no matter how good they were feeling. I believed what I had been taught in medical school, residency, and my gastroenterology training: that the only effective treatment for inflammatory bowel disease (IBD) was medication.

In 2004 I left full-time academics to open an integrative gastroenterology practice that incorporates the nutritional and lifestyle interventions I've come to believe in. I still carry a prescription pad, but I use it less and less often. Seeing patients for follow-up visits after they've instituted meaningful dietary and lifestyle changes, are feeling better, and no longer require medications are the victories I cherish. Our practice thrives on empowering people to improve their health in this simple and intuitive way: by nourishing themselves and their microbes, learning how to reduce stress, and incorporating more leisure into their daily lives.

What to Eat?

Many of the patients in our practice are on the Specific Carbohydrate Diet (SCD), a first cousin of the Paleo diet that allows some dairy in the form of do-it-yourself yogurt and aged cheeses but restricts cereals, grains, potatoes, and sugar. Others are strict Paleo devotees and committed to living a totally dairy- and grain-free life. Some avoid added sugar or sweeteners of any kind, while others use liberal amounts of raw honey or maple syrup. Most feel better when they eliminate dairy, and almost all agree that gluten is no good for their gut, but the amount and types of protein, fat, and carbohydrates they consume vary tremendously—from meat at every meal, to strict vegans. Once people figure out what dietary regimen works for them, some report that even a slight divergence leads to a flare-up of symptoms, while others are able to have "cheat days" once a week or still feel good when averaging about 80 percent compliance.

These observations led me to embark on the study I described in Chapter 3, which used dietary modification as the main therapeutic intervention in a group of patients with Crohn's disease and ulcerative colitis (see page 33). We used the results from the study as the basis for the advice we gave other patients in our practice, and the recommendations worked well not just for IBD but for many different types of gastrointestinal (GI) problems, especially those with disordered gut bacteria as the root cause. Our experience confirms what others have found: inflammation in the gut—and elsewhere in the body—can often be healed through dietary changes.

The idea that what you eat can affect what's going on in your gut, as well as the microbes that live there, may seem intuitive to you, but in conventional medical circles this is still a controversial notion. We've grown dependent on shortsighted pharmaceutical fixes, and the high cost we pay in side effects has become a familiar and accepted part of our medical landscape. Some of my colleagues seem downright baffled by the fact that I recommend cutting out junk food, eating lots of plants, taking probiotics, and incorporating stress-reducing techniques as the initial intervention for my Crohn's and ulcerative colitis patients, instead of prescribing medications associated with cancer and serious infection. One of the most common questions I'm asked is, "Does that stuff work?" It doesn't work for everyone. Some people have irreversible damage at a cellular level that doesn't respond to an integrative approach, and symptoms can be resistant even to heavy-duty pharmaceuticals. But most of the patients I treat respond extremely well to nutritional therapy, which makes sense now that we're aware of the relationship between a disordered microbiome and disease. Let's take a closer look at the specifics of the diet.

The Best of Both Worlds

A Paleo diet includes animal protein but excludes grains and legumes, while a vegan diet includes grains and legumes but excludes animal protein. Despite these striking differences, the healthiest versions of these two regimens have much more in common than you might think: they both encourage consumption of healthy plant-based foods such as fruits, vegetables, nuts, and seeds, and they exclude dairy products (which many people don't tolerate because they lack the enzyme to digest them and which are high in saturated fats, are ideally suited for baby cows, and in commercially available form don't do much for your microbiome since pasteurization kills off much of the beneficial bacteria).

The Live Dirty, Eat Clean Diet combines the best aspects of veganism and Paleo:

- Lots of high-fiber plant matter in the form of fresh vegetables and fruits
- Microbe-boosting whole grains and legumes that contain food for our microbes to eat

- The option of a small amount of high-quality protein and fat from animal sources

Like the Paleo diet, refined sugars and processed carbohydrates are not part of the approach, and like the vegan diet, the emphasis is on plants. It's a way of eating designed to feed your microbes, and it can help you get healthy and lose weight. It has helped hundreds of patients in my medical practice get relief from complaints of gas and bloating and has been a crucial part of my therapeutic approach to more severe forms of dysbiosis and serious autoimmune diseases such as Crohn's and ulcerative colitis.

The Veleo Approach

What I've just described is the way many health-conscious people eat without having a specific name to describe it, although some have called it a modified Paleo diet, or a "flexetarian" way of eating. Mark Hyman, MD, calls this cross between Paleo and vegan a "Pegan" diet, and he recommends it for diabetes, obesity, and the deadly combination of elevated cholesterol, high blood sugar levels, hypertension, and belly fat known as metabolic syndrome. I prefer the term *Veleo*, to emphasize the vegetable-based philosophy. Because a limited amount of animal products is allowed but not required, it's completely compatible with being a strict vegan, and Paleo followers are welcome to exclude grains or legumes if they feel better without them. But what's absolutely essential if you're trying to rehab your microbiome is large amounts of the type of plant fiber that isn't completely digested—leaving lots of leftovers to feed your microbes. These indigestible or poorly digestible fibers are the hallmark of the Live Dirty, Eat Clean Diet.

Before we delve into the specifics of what's included, excluded, and allowed in moderation, let's look at ten secrets for maximizing your success on the Live Dirty, Eat Clean Diet.

Success Secret #1: Choose Your Carbs Carefully

Many of us have been conditioned to think of carbohydrates as "bad" foods that make us fat and cause diabetes. But all carbs are definitely not created equal, and it's important to know which ones are actually good for your microbes and which ones you should avoid. Simple carbohydrates ("bad" carbs) found in soda, baked goods, and other processed grains are rapidly digested in the small intestine and absorbed as glucose, which produces about 4 calories of energy per gram digested. They cause a spike in insulin levels and are associated with weight gain, diabetes, and inflammation. They also cause undesirable shifts in microbial composition and can lead to the proliferation of yeast species.

Complex carbohydrates ("good" carbs) are typically high in fiber and include foods like fruits, vegetables, some whole grains, beans, and brown rice. Because of their high fiber content, these foods don't cause a surge in insulin levels and, from a microbial point of view, they're one of the most important foods for nurturing essential microbes. Here are some good carbs that are great for the microbiome that you should know about:

Resistant Starches

Resistant starches are a specific type of complex carbohydrate that don't get digested in the small intestine but rather travel through the GI tract relatively intact until they reach the colon, where they are fermented by gut bacteria to produce short-chain fatty acids (SCFAs). They contribute far fewer calories to our bottom line—only about 1.5 calories per gram compared to 4 calories per gram for simple carbohydrates. They're also good for the gut. SCFAs like butyrate are extremely important for colonic health: they're a primary energy source for colonic cells, they have anti-inflammatory and anticarcinogenic

TABLE 9-1 • Food High in Resistant Starches

- Green bananas
- Green banana flour
- Green peas
- Lentils
- Uncooked rolled oats
- White beans

properties, and they've been shown to increase colonic absorption of minerals.

Resistant starches function more like dietary fiber than starch, encouraging the growth of healthy microbes in the colon and acting as what is known as a prebiotic food: one that actually feeds gut bacteria and reduces production of potentially harmful compounds such as bile acids and ammonia (we'll talk more about prebiotics in Chapter 12). Green (unripe) bananas are my favorite resistant starch. You can eat them mashed instead of white potatoes, or substitute green banana flour for wheat flour in baked goods to help control weight, prevent a spike in your blood sugar, and reduce your risk for diabetes, while also helping your gut garden to flourish.

Inulin

Inulin is another type of complex carbohydrate known as a fructan. Like resistant starches, inulin also has prebiotic qualities: it feeds your microbes to promote a healthy gut flora. Adding inulin-containing foods such as leeks to soups or stews, ripe bananas to your green smoothies, and garlic and onion for sautéing whatever you're cooking can help to increase the amount of inulin in your diet.

TABLE 9–2 • Foods High in Inulin

- Artichokes
- Asparagus
- Bananas
- Chicory root
- Dandelion root
- Garlic
- Leeks
- Onions

Success Secret #2: Ferment Your Food

Fermented foods such as sauerkraut, kimchi, and pickles are microbiome rock stars because they contain live bacteria (probiotics) *and* prebiotic fiber to nourish gut bacteria. You should try to include some of these fermented foods in your diet every day. They're super-easy to make—mostly involving just adding a little sea salt and some water to veggies—and after fermenting, they can keep in your refrigerator for weeks. You'll find delicious recipes and step-by-step instructions for fermenting various foods in the Recipes section at the end of this book.

Success Secret #3: Manage Your Meat Intake

Italian researcher Paolo Lionetti compared children eating a fiber-rich, plant-based diet consisting of mostly legumes and vegetables with those on a high-fat/high-sugar diet that included lots of animal protein. The results revealed vast differences in gut bacteria: the high-fat/high-sugar group had less microbial diversity and more species associated with allergies, diarrhea, and obesity, while the high-fiber group had higher levels of beneficial SCFAs that protect against inflammation and more species associated with leanness.

Could sugar consumption alone have caused the undesirable microbial profile in the high-fat/high-sugar group? A recent study suggests otherwise. Harvard scientists put a group of nine volunteers on two extreme diets for five days each. The first diet was a high-fat, low-fiber regimen with lots of animal protein that included brisket, salami, prosciutto, and an assortment of cheeses. The second diet was a low-fat, high-fiber vegan diet that included jasmine rice, onions, tomatoes, squash, peas, lentils, and garlic, with bananas and mangoes for snacks. The scientists analyzed the study participants' microbiomes before, during, and after each diet. The differences were apparent much more quickly than anyone anticipated and had unexpected genetic consequences. Not only did the relative numbers of the various gut bacteria start to shift within a day—bile-loving species that help break down fat but have been associated with inflammation and colitis dominated during the meat and cheese diet—but the genes that were turned on changed, too.

Extremely low-carb diets, especially those that restrict carbohydrates to less than 50 grams daily, can result in too little dietary fiber and a microbial profile with decreased species diversity, similar to what we observe after people take antibiotics. Bottom line: it's not that meat is necessarily bad for the microbiome; it's that dietary fiber is good for it, and eating too much of the former can lead to not eating enough of the latter.

There's only so much room on your plate, and it's vitally important to make sure that the microbe-boosting foods are well represented. So ideally, you should think of the veggies as the main course and meat as a condiment. Make sure you're eating the best-quality, grass-fed meat available, with no antibiotics, since cows raised on corn or treated with antibiotics produce more pathogenic bacteria, such as *E. coli* 0157:H7, that can disrupt the microbiome and cause serious illness in humans.

The amount of meat you eat can alter the composition of the microbiome, but the microbiome also has an effect on the meat you consume. Research from the Cleveland Clinic shows that when gut bacteria ingest L-carnitine, a compound found in red meat, they can convert it into a chemical called TMAO (trimethylamine N-oxide) that's associated with artery-clogging plaque formation. So gut bacteria may be intimately involved with the heart attacks and strokes associated with the high consumption of red meat. Interestingly, when vegans and vegetarians consume L-carnitine, they don't produce nearly as much TMAO, likely because of differences in gut bacteria from eating a plant-based diet. Other foods such as poultry, eggs, seafood, pork, and dairy also contain L-carnitine, but red meat has the highest amount.

What's also worth considering when deciding how much, if any, animal protein should be part of your microbial plan, is the fact that raising animals for human consumption is hard on the environment, and even harder on the animals raised in conditions of pain and suffering. When it comes to the microbiome, plants are where it's at. For that reason, plus the reasons above, you might consider cutting your animal intake way down, or even forgoing it altogether.

Success Secret #4: Eat More Plants

One can argue about the merits of eating or not eating meat when it comes to the microbiome, but there's no debate that eating more plants is the most important strategy for improving gut flora. Indigestible dietary fiber from plants provides the raw material for bacterial fermentation, which feeds your microbes and produces health-promoting SCFAs. The diversity and number of plants you eat will be reflected in the diversity and number of bacteria you grow in your gut garden, so you need to eat lots of different plants every day.

Not eating enough indigestible plant matter to nourish your microbes is one of the most common reasons dysbiosis may not get better when people adopt a Paleo or low-carb lifestyle. Vegetables are the least commonly consumed food in the American diet, and the most important when it comes to microbial health—which is why the Live Dirty, Eat Clean Diet focuses so much on consuming them, and why it recommends limiting animal protein and fat. A helpful way to think about the relationship between eating plants and gut bacteria is that the plant fiber that can't be broken down and absorbed by your body ends up feeding your colonic bacteria instead. That means less food for you (think easier weight loss) and more for your microbes! The tough fibrous part of plants, like the stems of broccoli or the base of asparagus, provide the most indigestible fiber, so you need to make sure you're eating the whole plant.

When we don't eat enough plant fiber, we risk starving the essential bacteria we're trying to cultivate. According to researcher Jeff Leach, founder of the Human Food Project, when there are inadequate amounts of dietary fiber around, gut bacteria can start eating us instead—breaking down the protective mucinous lining of our intestine. Well-fed bacteria, on the other hand, produce nutrients like SCFAs that nourish the intestinal cells.

Success Secret #5: Choose Food with Dirt on It

The main difference between the produce you buy at the supermarket and what you find at most farm stands is dirt and distance. These days, our produce travels long distances—sometimes thousands of miles from other continents—before it gets to us. The enzymatic activity and nutrient value of these foods starts to decline right after harvesting, and therefore its microbial value is significantly diminished. Buying locally grown food from small farmers generally means that the food has traveled a shorter distance to get to you, so more of the nutrients and bacteria are intact. You'll probably find that it stays fresh longer, too.

Chances are also higher that it's been grown in small batches in soil, rather than in the aseptic factory environment of mass-produced food. Look for produce that has evidence of dirt on it (although you still need to wash it before you eat it), and that isn't perfectly uniform in color or size, reflecting the normal variation of food grown in nature, rather than engineered to look a certain way. And of course, organically produced food, grown with dirt rather than chemicals, is always best.

Success Secret #6: Say No to Sugar

Sugar feeds gut bacteria—but not the kind whose growth you want to encourage. Studies have shown that a diet high in sugar can lead to overgrowth of yeast species and other pathogenic bacteria. As I described in Chapter 5, sugar is often habit-forming because it increases the microbial populations that thrive on it, which then increase your cravings for more sugar. Whether you gradually reduce your sugar consumption or do a more drastic sugar detox, your gut bacteria should eventually get to the point where the sugar-craving microbes are outnumbered and your cravings become easier to control.

Sugar interferes with the ability of our white blood cells to destroy toxins—an effect that starts within minutes of eating it and can last for several hours. So, in addition to causing imbalance in your microbiome, sugar can actually impair your body's ability to fight infection. Honey has a lower glycemic index than regular sugar, which means it releases less glucose into the bloodstream, and in some studies it has been described as having prebiotic properties, so it's a reasonable alternative to sugar (although if you suffer from severe forms of dysbiosis, including yeast overgrowth, you may want to use honey more sparingly). High-nutrient raw versions such as manuka honey are what I recommend. As you'll see in Chapter 10, it can also be used on your body as a wonderful addition to your skin care regimen.

Artificial sweeteners are just as bad, if not worse, for your microbiome than their natural counterparts. Recent research suggests that they cause changes in gut bacteria that promote glucose intolerance, making them a major risk factor for developing diabetes.

Success Secret #7: Focus on Addition Instead of Subtraction

When my friends and patients complain about their kids (or spouses) being picky eaters, I try to get them to focus more on making healthy additions to their plates rather than on the not-so-healthy foods they need to get rid of. It's the absence of nourishing food rather than the presence of the not-so-good stuff that usually leads to a depleted microbiome. For most of us, eating enough asparagus and leeks, to name two examples, can balance out a slice of cake here and there. That's why the Live Dirty, Eat Clean Diet emphasizes dietary fiber—the preferred food for essential bacteria—above all else. If we can get our picky eaters to add in more good stuff, we can crowd out the less helpful foods, even if we don't eliminate them altogether.

Success Secret #8: Retrain the Taste Buds

Gradually training the taste buds to accept more bitter-tasting greens and cutting down on intake of added sugar are key elements of retraining a picky palate. And you really should think of this as training—it can take months, if not years, for people to get to the point where they're eating vegetables at every meal without rebelling, or enjoying more savory rather than sweet desserts. It's also important to remember that food is medicine: you're not really feeding your picky eater; you're feeding his or her microbes to safeguard against future diseases.

Here are some of my favorite strategies for retraining the taste buds and getting more plant fiber onto the plate:

- Substitute:
  - zucchini "noodles" for wheat pasta
  - roasted squash or sweet potato for french fries
  - mashed green bananas for mashed potatoes
  - mashed cauliflower for white rice
- Add in:
  - spinach and kale to smoothies
  - leeks and celery to soups and stews

- roasted pumpkin or squash instead of flour to thicken sauces
- onions, garlic, peppers, and spinach to scrambled eggs
- Reduce sweetness with:
  - frozen bananas blended with almond butter "ice cream"
  - dates filled with nut butter to satisfy sugar cravings
  - raw honey instead of sugar when baking, and halve the amount called for in the recipe
  - fresh ginger instead of sugar in herbal tea or lemonade

Success Secret #9: Eliminate Franken Foods and Friends

Eliminating foods that have been modified and adulterated from what nature intended is good for your microbiome for a number of reasons: they may have additives and preservatives that can be harmful to gut bacteria; they may be full of hormones; they may contain detectable levels of antibiotics; they may have been sprayed with pesticides that are toxic to our microbiome; they may be genetically modified "Franken foods" that our GI tracts have a hard time digesting; most of the healthy fiber may have been removed during processing; or they may not provide enough nutrients to encourage the growth of healthy bacteria. Foods like gluten, dairy, refined carbohydrates, processed foods in general, GMO foods, and artificial sweeteners all fit the bill.

Success Secret #10: Follow My 1-2-3 Rule

I'm not a fan of counting calories, rationing carbohydrates, keeping track of grams of protein, or anything else that tries to turn the art, pleasure, and comfort of eating into too much of a scientific endeavor. But there is one simple rule I strongly recommend. I call it my 1-2-3 Rule:

> ## My 1-2-3 Rule
>
> Eat at least one vegetable at breakfast, two at lunch, and three at dinner.

There are many ways to accomplish this. It could be a smoothie with kale or a spinach omelet for breakfast, salad with chopped raw veggies for lunch, and steamed asparagus plus a salad of lettuce and cucumbers with your dinner. The 1-2-3 Rule is a great way to make sure you're getting enough dietary fiber without getting bogged down in too many details, and focusing on building your meal around plants will help you think about meat as a side dish rather than the main event—a great microbe-boosting strategy. Fermented foods can be eaten as a condiment with any meal and have a double benefit: they'll count toward your 1-2-3 goals while also providing additional bacteria themselves.

The Live Dirty, Eat Clean Diet

Now that you know the secrets for success on the Live Dirty, Eat Clean Diet, let's profile the foods in your day-to-day diet in more detail. In line with my goal of keeping eating easy and pleasurable, I've divided the food lists below into three types: green light foods, which you can eat as much as you like; yellow light foods, which I recommend you limit to one small (four-ounce) serving a day; and red light foods, which should be avoided or reduced, depending on your health issues and goals in general and your gut health in particular.

Green Light Foods

Most of these foods contain indigestible plant fiber that nourishes the microbiome. Others have healthy fats such as omega-3 fatty acids that have anti-inflammatory properties. Some may not have specific microbe-boosting features but can be enjoyed without any ill effects on gut bacteria. You can eat as many of these foods as you need to feel full—don't worry about calories or portion size! Be sure to include plenty of prebiotic foods such as onions, garlic, leeks, artichokes, beans, asparagus, carrots, radishes, tomatoes, bananas, ground raw flaxseeds, bitter greens such as radicchio, and chicory, as well as fermented foods such as sauerkraut and kimchi.

- Fruits
- Vegetables
- Root vegetables
- Nuts
- Nut butters
- Seeds
- Legumes (beans, peas, peanuts, chickpeas)
- Olive oil
- Coconut oil
- Organic raw honey
- Brown rice
- Sweet potato
- Squash
- Quinoa
- Oats (steel-cut or old-fashioned gluten-free oats)
- Unsweetened dried fruits

Green Light Drinks

- Water
- Carbonated water
- Unsweetened, unflavored coconut water
- Dairy substitutes: almond milk, hemp milk, cashew milk, coconut milk (unsweetened)

- Herbal tea
- Smoothies (with no added sugar or sweeteners)
- Vegetable juices (with no added sugar or sweeteners)

Green Light Baking

- Almond flour
- Coconut flour
- Chickpea flour
- Brown rice flour
- Green banana flour

Yellow Light Foods

These foods aren't specifically beneficial to the microbiome, but they can be enjoyed in moderation without any deleterious effects. I recommend that you limit your consumption to one serving (approximately four ounces) daily. Organic, antibiotic-free animal products are best.

- 1 serving per day of animal protein
  - Wild fish
  - Wild game
  - Grass-fed beef
  - Organic meat/poultry/eggs
- Ghee/clarified butter
- No more than 1 serving per day of alcohol

Red Light Foods

When consumed regularly, these foods are associated with dysbiosis, either because they're broken down into simple sugars upon digestion, are highly processed, or contain ingredients that damage the intestinal lining or the microbes that live there.

- Dairy (except ghee/clarified butter)
- Sugar (organic raw honey allowed)
- Artificial sweeteners (aspartame, stevia, sorbitol, mannitol, etc.)
- High fructose corn syrup
- Corn/corn products
- Gluten
- Grains (except brown rice)
- White rice
- White potato
- Pasta (except brown rice pasta or quinoa pasta that does not contain corn)
- Processed carbohydrates
- Refined oils (canola, safflower, etc.)
- Sodas
- Diet sodas
- Fruit juices

You Are What Your Gut Bacteria Eat

What you eat has a more profound impact on your microbiome than anything else you do. The good news is that microbial health is based on the sum total of what you eat, not on any one ingredient or food group. The Live Dirty, Eat Clean Diet is a safe and effective way to rehab your microbiome and holds real promise if you're suffering from dysbiosis or simply looking to improve your health and lower your risk of developing disease.

CHAPTER 10

||||||||||||||||||||||||||||||||||||||||

The Live Dirty Lifestyle

ODERN HUMANS spend 90 percent of their time indoors—in buildings or in vehicles with closed windows and doors that limit contact with nature and afford little opportunity for re-wilding. Studies show that as the amount of concrete and glass in a neighborhood increases, the diversity of microbial species on people's skin decreases, and their risk for allergies and asthma goes up.

Harsh cleansers and antibacterial products super-sanitize our bodies and our already sterile environment, threatening the existence of what few microbes remain, and our overscheduled lives leave little time to get outside and literally smell the roses. Most of us live in small, clean clusters rather than in large extended family households, so we don't have the benefit of swapping microbes with cousins, aunties, and uncles.

If we want to invigorate our lackluster microbiome and improve our health, we need to figure out how to escape the microbial discord of our modern existence and get back to a slightly dirtier, healthier way of life. Here are some ways to embrace a little grime and grow some microbes at the same time.

It's OK to Be a Little Dirty

When it comes to your appearance, your microbes might actually play a bigger role than your genes, because without a healthy microbiome, it's really hard to have glowing skin or a full head of hair. Your gut bacteria are like the soil, and your hair and skin are like the plants. If the soil is unhealthy because of too many chemicals and not enough of the right nutrients, the plants won't bloom properly.

Chemicals such as sodium lauryl sulfate are common ingredients in cleansing products because they create a thick lather, but they're also easily absorbed and very irritating to your skin. Harsh chemicals like these make your skin and scalp more permeable to penetration by surface bacteria and viruses, as well as to other chemicals, creating a state of dysbiosis and putting you at risk for developing skin conditions such as acne, eczema, and rosacea.

Bacteria that metabolize ammonia, known as ammonia-oxidizing bacteria, or AOB, are found in soil and untreated water and play an important role in the recycling of nitrogen (an essential element of all life on earth), and maybe in the health of our skin. In a small study of volunteers, the group using a suspension of live AOB on their face and scalp noted significant improvements in their skin compared to the group using a placebo. These were subjective findings, but ongoing studies are examining the effectiveness of AOB and other topically applied microbes as treatments for acne, eczema, and other skin conditions. How ironic that the treatment for acne may actually be adding more microbes to the skin rather than removing them, as so many acne preparations do.

David Whitlock, the founder of a company that isolates AOB for commercial use, hasn't showered since 2002, although he does take the occasional sponge bath, and he douses himself with AOB regularly. Other converts to this idea of skipping soap in favor of a more au naturel approach frequently report healthier skin and hair and—

perhaps not surprisingly, given what I'm going to share with you about armpits later in this chapter—fewer problems with body odor. Whitlock hypothesizes that the reason horses and other large mammals roll around in the dirt, especially when they're hot and sweaty, is to acquire more AOB that can metabolize ammonia, one of the main ingredients in sweat.

The dirt on your body doesn't need cleansing any more than the microbes inside you do. Most of us aren't rolling around in the mud (which might not actually be such a bad idea), so we hardly need to be washing our skin and hair every day, stripping away the oils and bacteria that keep them healthy, and replacing them with inferior store-bought versions. Just as formula can never be as good as breast milk, so there's no synthetic product you can apply to your skin or hair that can improve on what your own body can produce.

It's OK to Be a Little Sweaty

You probably know that exercise is good for you, but it turns out it's also really good for your microbes. A 2014 British study compared stool samples from professional rugby players in the midst of their training season to those of healthy men of the same age who weren't avid exercisers. The athletes' stool samples had more bacteria, greater species diversity, and significantly higher levels of the species that are associated with low rates of obesity and obesity-related diseases. The rugby players also ate a lot more fruit and vegetables. The study authors concluded that "exercise seems to be another important factor in the relationship between the microbiota, host immunity and host metabolism, with diet playing an important role."

Exercise also stimulates peristalsis in your gut, which keeps the products of digestion moving and can help prevent small intestinal bacterial overgrowth (SIBO). You don't need to be a professional rugby player to benefit from the microbe-boosting effects of exercise. Simply elevating your heart rate to 20 percent above baseline with a brisk walk for thirty minutes three to five times a week is enough to stimulate peristalsis. And try not bathing afterward to enhance the effect!

It's OK to Have a Little B.O.

The two main types of bacteria that inhabit your armpits are *Staphylococci* and *Corynebacterium*. *Staph* tends to be the dominant species in women and has very little smell, while more odor-producing *Corynebacterium* predominates in men, probably because they secrete more fat in their sweat, which is the preferred food of lipid-loving *Corynebacterium*. A Belgian study confirmed what I have long suspected: the more antiperspirant you use, the more you need. Aluminum salts in antiperspirants have a greater impact on *Staph*, disproportionately depleting their numbers, which leads to an increase in the population of smelly *Corynebacterium*. So, when you use these products, you're actually altering the microbiome of your armpit—and not for the better. (Vaginal douching is a similarly bad idea that not only begets more douching but also decreases the native protective *Lactobacillus* population and increases the risk of sexually transmitted diseases and urinary tract infections. Remember, you're not supposed to smell like a bouquet of flowers.)

If quitting antiperspirants cold turkey seems a bit too drastic, then consider using less and try going without on days when you're not working closely alongside others, or dab a few drops of lavender essential oil under your armpits. Pungent bacteria from your skin grow more readily on synthetic fabrics such as polyester, so wearing clothes made from natural fabrics like cotton or linen can help with odor control. Attitudes toward body odor vary across cultures, and it might be helpful to follow the lead of other societies where there's more acceptance toward having a discernible personal odor. It may take a little getting used to, but noses do acclimate to sensing our more natural smells.

When my daughter entered middle school, I noticed she had more body odor at the end of soccer practice or after an active day at school. This feral scent that for millennia has helped animals—and humans— in the wild recognize each other now seems to be a major social liability. She was completely unbothered by it, but I found myself constantly smelling her armpits. I ultimately did what I recommend you do: stop sniffing around so much and remember that smelly is in the nose of the beholder.

How Chilling Out and Changing Your Diet Can Make You Smell Better

There's a fascinating connection among stress, microbes, and body odor. You have two kinds of sweat glands: eccrine glands, which are located all over your body and open to the skin, and apocrine glands, which release their contents into areas with hair follicles like your armpits and groin. Eccrine glands secrete odorless water and salt onto your skin when it's hot or when you're exercising, which helps cool you off as it evaporates. Apocrine glands release a milky white substance when you're stressed that combines with bacteria in your armpits and groin to create smelly body odor. Most people can clearly distinguish between the slightly salty smell they have after a hard workout or on a hot day and the mustier smell of being stressed out—all the more reason to hone your relaxation response if you want to feel (and smell) like a bed of roses.

Stress may make you smelly, but the scents emanating from your body are also a reflection of what you're putting into it. The unfortunate cows that are fed corn in the feedlot tend to have malodorous stool and gas as a result of the difference in bacterial populations (more pathogenic microbes like *E. coli*) that an unnatural diet like corn, instead of grass, produces. We suffer the same misfortune when it comes to our own body odor, stool, and gas when we eat an unnatural diet full of processed grains instead of fresh fruits and vegetables. A change in your personal aroma is one of the first things you'll start to notice as your microbiome shifts and gets healthier. The nose knows!

TABLE 10–1 • Live Dirty Lifestyle Dos

- DO use a chlorine filter for the water you bathe with and drink.
- DO use just water and no soap when you bathe.
- If you're really filthy or not ready to give up soap, DO stick to mild nonbacterial ones made from organic nonsynthetic oils and use them sparingly just in moist areas like the groin and under the arms, not on the rest of your skin.
- DO get a bidet so you can rinse your nooks and crannies without having to wash your whole body.
- DO cleanse your scalp with essential oils or with diluted apple cider vinegar instead of shampoo (see Rinse for Oily Hair, page 149, and Essential Oil Scalp Treatment, page 149).
- DO use a natural conditioning mask made from coconut oil and avocado if you have dry hair (see Moisturizing Hair Mask for Dry/Damaged Hair, page 148).
- DO use scents made from essential oils instead of alcohol.
- DO use edible hair and skin products and make them yourself (see my recipes at the end of this chapter).
- DO get sweaty—people who exercise regularly have greater diversity of gut bacteria.
- DO consider getting a dog, cat, rabbit, or other pet: children with pets have fewer infections and require fewer antibiotics.
- DO let your children get dirty, play on the ground, and be around other kids (good for grown-ups, too).
- DO get your hands dirty by starting a garden. Exposing your immune system to the trillions of microbes in soil is a great way to literally grow a good gut garden.
- DO open your windows. Letting nature in will improve the health and diversity of the microbes in your home.
- DO fill your house with plants for additional microbial exposure.
- DO make your own natural household cleaner by mixing ½ cup white vinegar with 4 cups of water, 12 drops of tea tree oil, and 12 drops of lavender essential oil. Combine the ingredients in a spray bottle and shake well before using.

TABLE 10–2 • Live Dirty Lifestyle Don'ts

- DON'T use things *on* your body that you wouldn't put *in* your body. Stick to skin- and hair-care products with edible food grade ingredients (see my recipes at the end of this chapter).
- DON'T bathe more frequently than every other day unless you're really filthy.
- DON'T use soaps, cleansers, or moisturizers that contain petroleum products, FD&C dyes, fragrances, parabens, phthalates, sodium lauryl sulfate, sodium laureth sulfate, triclosan, triethylamine, or other harmful chemicals.
- DON'T shampoo your hair more than once a week, and avoid shampoos with detergents such as sodium lauryl sulfate or sodium laureth sulfate, which can make your skin and scalp more sensitive and permeable to toxins.
- DON'T use scents containing alcohol that can harm skin microbes.
- DON'T use hand sanitizer.
- DON'T use antibacterial soaps and products.
- DON'T use antiperspirants—they can alter your skin microbiome.
- DON'T use mouthwash—it can destroy the microbial ecosystem in your mouth.
- DON'T use chemical household cleaners (see my recipe on page 144).

Beauty Products That Are Good for You and Your Microbes

Coconut oil is the main ingredient in the hair and skin products I create at home. It makes a great moisturizer, makeup remover, exfoliator, hair conditioner, massage oil, personal lubricant, and lip balm—and it's great in the kitchen, too. Coconut oil has antifungal properties and can also inhibit the growth of bad bacteria, while its healthy fats moisturize and nourish the skin. When warming coconut oil to room temperature, use very gentle heat or rub it between your palms to get it to a more liquid consistency. Raw, unrefined, virgin, organic coconut oil is best.

Manuka honey is produced from bees that feed on the manuka tree, which is native to Australia and New Zealand. It's been used medicinally to help with skin healing in cases of superficial burns, and it has some natural properties that can protect against skin pathogens. Most important, it won't disrupt the normal pH of your skin or harm essential microbial species, so it makes a great base for skin cleansers and body scrubs. It's the only thing I use to wash my face, and it has helped keep my rosacea under control.

Edible Recipes for Skin and Hair

Your skin is a porous membrane that absorbs or "eats" what you put on it, which can have a profound effect on both your internal microbiome and your external microbiome. I recommend applying the same philosophy to your skin and hair care that you follow in the kitchen: use high-quality, simple ingredients such as raw honey, papaya, oatmeal, and coconut oil straight from nature, not from the laboratory. Here are some of my favorite beauty recipes.

Oily Skin Facial Scrub

2 tablespoons manuka honey

1 tablespoon oatmeal

1½ teaspoons cornmeal

1 teaspoon lemon juice

✳ MOISTEN YOUR FACE AND HANDS with water and mix all of the ingredients in the palms of your hands. Gently rub the paste all over your face in a circular motion for 1 minute. The cornmeal and lemon juice are great natural exfoliants, but if you apply too much pressure or scrub too hard, you can irritate your skin.

Wash off with lukewarm water and a clean wet washcloth. Can be used once per week. Make a larger batch to use on the rest of your body.

Dry Skin Facial Scrub

2 tablespoons manuka honey

2 tablespoons fresh ripe papaya (skin and seeds removed)

1 tablespoon oatmeal

✳ MOISTEN YOUR FACE AND HANDS with water and mix all of the ingredients in the palms of your hands. Gently rub the paste all over your face and neck in a circular motion. Massage for 1 to 2 minutes. Wash off with lukewarm water and a clean wet washcloth. Can be used once per week. Make a larger batch to use on the rest of your body.

Coconut Oil Exfoliating/Moisturizing Body Scrub

4 tablespoons manuka honey

2 tablespoons coconut oil

1 tablespoon ground psyllium husk or cornmeal

✳ MOISTEN YOUR BODY AND HANDS with water and mix all of the ingredients in the palms of your hands. Gently rub the paste all over your body, paying special attention to any rough patches of skin. Wash off with lukewarm water and a clean wet washcloth. Can be used daily.

Warm Brown Sugar Exfoliating/ Moisturizing Body Scrub

3 tablespoons coconut oil

2 tablespoons brown sugar

2 tablespoons manuka honey

1 tablespoon pure vanilla extract

✳ IN A SMALL PAN, combine all of the ingredients and heat gently until the coconut oil is completely liquid and the brown sugar has dissolved. Mix well. Allow the paste to cool to a comfortable temperature. Then gently massage it all over your body. Wash off with lukewarm water and a clean wet washcloth. Can be used daily.

Vanilla Moisturizing Lotion

4 tablespoons coconut oil
½ teaspoon pure vanilla extract

✳ MIX THE COCONUT OIL and vanilla well in the palms of your hands or in a small bowl and apply liberally all over your body. Can be used daily.

Moisturizing Citrus Lotion

4 tablespoons coconut oil
½ teaspoon orange or lemon zest

✳ MIX THE COCONUT OIL and orange zest well in the palms of your hands or in a small bowl and apply liberally all over your body. Can be used daily.

Moisturizing Hair Mask for Dry/Damaged Hair

2 tablespoons coconut oil
1 tablespoon olive oil
1 ripe avocado, pitted and peeled

✳ IN A SMALL BOWL, combine all of the ingredients and mix well to form a paste. Apply the paste to wet hair, working it through from the roots to the ends. Wrap your hair in a warm towel or plastic wrap and leave the paste in for a minimum of 30 minutes or as long as overnight. Rinse well with lukewarm water. Do not shampoo or condition your hair afterward. Use once a month.

Rinse for Oily Hair

1 cup apple cider vinegar

1 cup water

✳ IN A BOWL, combine the apple cider vinegar and water. Apply to wet hair, working it through from the roots to the ends and massaging it into the scalp. Leave in for 5 minutes and then rinse with water. Do not shampoo or condition your hair afterward. Use once a month. May strip color if your hair is colored with hair dye or henna.

Essential Oil Scalp Treatment

1 teaspoon therapeutic-grade organic or wild-crafted lavender or other essential oil

✳ PART YOUR HAIR INTO four or more sections to allow better access to the scalp. Moisten your fingertips with essential oil and massage your scalp vigorously for 2 to 3 minutes. Rinse your scalp with water. Do not shampoo or condition your hair afterward.

Getting Rid of the Chemicals

I've been reading nutrition labels at the grocery store for years, but after my daughter was born I started paying more attention to the labels on personal care products such as the shampoos and lotions that I was using on both her and myself, and the cleaners we used every day in our home. I was shocked when I researched the side effects of some of the ingredients (the Environmental Working Group database is a great resource) and was struck by the similarities between those products and what was passing for food in the supermarket: full of potentially harmful chemicals, cheap to manufacture, and a long shelf life. Surely what I was using on my body and in my home had important consequences for my microbiome? My personal challenges with eczema and rosacea were what inspired me to gather up all the shampoos, soaps, conditioners, perfumes, lotions, household cleaners, and detergents with ingredients whose names I couldn't pronounce, and replace them with simple homemade versions made with things like vinegar, honey, lemon, and essential oils.

If you struggle with dysbiosis, changing your diet and taking a good probiotic may not be enough. You may be destroying essential microbes every day with the products you use. When you let go of preconceived notions of cleanliness and personal hygiene that have more to do with aggressive marketing than health, and really embrace the idea of germs as friends rather than foes, a new paradigm starts to emerge that's based on peaceful coexistence and synergy rather than toxic extermination. So go ahead, get a little dirty. Your microbiome will thank you.

CHAPTER 11

||||||||||||||||||||||||||||||||||||||||||||

A Rewilding
Approach to Illness

A S A PHYSICIAN, I realize I have inside knowledge that makes it easier for me to decide whether an antibiotic or a trip to the doctor is truly necessary, and in no way am I advocating that you stop taking medication or delay seeking advice from a health professional when you're sick. But I am advocating that you become the kind of patient who analyzes and queries medical advice, and engages your health care professional in respectful dialogue that may include some pointed questions. Conventional medicine is finally beginning to embrace the importance of the microbiome and the role it plays in human health, but not all practitioners—or consumers—are equally enlightened. Many still consider antibiotics to be a reasonable course of action with limited downside for the treatment of minor illnesses.

In this chapter, I'll share some critical questions to ask your health care provider if you've been prescribed an antibiotic, tell you which microbe-harming drugs are best avoided, provide you with some health tips to protect your microbes, outline alternative approaches to illness that may help you avoid antibiotics, and offer a sample birth plan to ensure that your baby is born with his or her full complement of microbes.

TABLE 11–1 • Ten Questions for Your Health Care Provider If You've Been Prescribed an Antibiotic

The first question on this list is the most important, and while it may not be necessary to go through all ten with your doctor, this list can help frame your conversation and indicate to whomever is doing the prescribing that you're not keen on taking an antibiotic unless absolutely necessary. Studies in both children and adults have shown that doctors are far more likely to prescribe an antibiotic when they perceive that the patient is interested in taking one, and there's generally a lot of leeway in whether antibiotic treatment is really needed.

1. Is the antibiotic prescribed for me absolutely necessary?
2. Is the antibiotic prescribed being used to treat an actual infection, or to prevent one?
3. Do you have the results of the culture, swab, or biopsy back yet that demonstrate an infection, or are you treating me presumptively because you think the results will be positive?
4. What other options are there for me to feel better besides an antibiotic?
5. What would be the natural course of my illness if I didn't take an antibiotic?
6. How long should it take for me to start feeling better if I don't take an antibiotic?
7. If I do have to take an antibiotic, what's the shortest amount of time I can take it for?
8. Is there a more narrow-spectrum antibiotic such as penicillin that would still be effective for my condition?
9. If I decide not to take an antibiotic, what are the signs to watch for that might suggest that my condition is worsening and I might need to start an antibiotic?
10. What's the worst thing that could happen if I don't take an antibiotic?

TABLE 11–2 • Ten Things to Do When Taking Antibiotics

So you've voiced your desire to avoid antibiotics and queried your health care provider about whether they're absolutely necessary, but the verdict is in: a course of antibiotics is definitely warranted. Now what? Although it's true that your microbiome will take a hit and may be permanently altered, it's still possible to mitigate the damage by supporting your gut and your microbes during and after antibiotics. These ten tips will help minimize microbial loss and encourage rapid regrowth.

1. Take a probiotic during and after antibiotics. Several studies have documented the usefulness of probiotics in decreasing side effects such as antibiotic-associated diarrhea (AAD) and *Clostridium difficile* (*C. diff*), as well as repopulating the gut. You should start the probiotic at the same time you start the antibiotic, but try to take the probiotic dose at a time as far away from the antibiotics as possible. So, for example, if you're taking an antibiotic twice daily at 8:00 a.m. and 8:00 p.m., you would take the probiotic at 2:00 p.m. You also need to continue the probiotic for at least one month after finishing the course of antibiotics. Probiotics containing various strains of *Lactobacillus* and *Bifidobacteria* are the most useful, as well as those containing strains of the beneficial yeast *Saccharomyces boulardii* (500 mg daily), which is especially helpful in preventing *C. diff* and which isn't susceptible to antibiotics. See Chapter 12, "Bugs over Drugs: Probiotics and Other Supplements," for how to choose the right probiotic.

2. Request a narrow-spectrum antibiotic. Taking a narrow-spectrum antibiotic will minimize damage to your microbiome by targeting a narrower range of bacteria. Culture and sensitivity results from urine, stool, sputum, blood, skin, or other body parts, depending on the type and location of infection, will reveal which bacteria are present and which antibiotics they're

sensitive to, allowing your doctor to pick a narrow-spectrum antibiotic that will still be effective, rather than a broad-spectrum one that will needlessly kill off additional nonpathogenic bacteria. Having the culture results before starting antibiotic therapy ensures that the infection you're being treated for is actually sensitive to the antibiotic you're taking, which will help avoid retreatment with additional courses of antibiotics.

3. Eat prebiotic foods to support your microbiome. Foods high in fiber and resistant starch are especially important when you're taking an antibiotic. Not only do they provide food for your microbes, but they also help to promote species diversity, which can decrease dramatically after a course of antibiotics. Fermented foods such as sauerkraut and kimchi (see Sauerkraut, page 269, and Kimchi, page 264) feed your gut bacteria as well as provide additional live microbes themselves. See Chapter 9, "The Live Dirty, Eat Clean Diet," for a guide to the most important prebiotic foods, and follow my 1-2-3 rule to make sure you're getting several servings of microbe-boosting plant-based fiber each day.

4. Eliminate sugary, starchy foods. Deleting these foods from your diet is an essential part of rehabbing your microbiome, and it's particularly important when you're taking an antibiotic. Foods (and drinks) high in sugar and starchy foods that are broken down into simple sugars in the gut send undesirable yeast species into a feeding frenzy, further contributing to microbial imbalance induced by the antibiotics. If you're prone to yeast infections, following a strict anti-yeast diet that excludes any and all sugar while taking antibiotics and for thirty days afterward may be advisable.

5. Eat lots of yeast-fighting foods. Antibiotics are the main cause of yeast overgrowth, which can cause vaginal infections and lots of other symptoms (see Chapter 5 "Dysbiosis—Do You Have It?"). Foods with significant anti-yeast properties include onion, garlic, seaweed, rutabaga, pumpkin seeds, and coconut oil.

Make sure you're incorporating lots of these foods into your diet while taking antibiotics.

6. Drink ginger tea. Ginger has a soothing effect on the digestive system and can help to reduce gas and bloating associated with taking an antibiotic. For best results, peel a one-inch piece of fresh ginger root and cut it into small pieces and place in a teapot or thermal carafe. Then add two cups of boiling water and let steep for twenty to thirty minutes. Strain and serve.

7. Use bentonite. Medicinal clay has been used as far back as ancient Mesopotamia. Bentonite can help treat AAD by thickening stool, and it also has antibacterial (*E. coli* and *Staphylococcus aureus*) and antifungal (*Candida albicans*) effects. Use one tablespoon of bentonite clay (mixed with one tablespoon of unsweetened applesauce, if desired, for taste) one to two times daily until symptoms of AAD are alleviated. Be sure to separate the clay from the antibiotic and probiotic doses to avoid binding them and reducing their efficacy. Stop using the clay if constipation develops.

8. Make a mushroom tea. Shiitake and maitake mushrooms have been used as medicine by various cultures throughout the world for thousands of years. They have significant immune-boosting properties and antifungal effects. Chop two dried mushroom caps into small pieces. Add them to a small kettle or pot of water (about four cups) and bring to a boil. Reduce heat, cover, and simmer for about thirty minutes. Strain and serve. You can drink this mushroom tea daily while you're taking antibiotics.

9. Support your liver. Antibiotics, like most drugs, are broken down in the liver, so it's important to make sure that your liver is as healthy as possible while taking a course of antibiotics in order to avoid liver damage. Dark green leafy vegetables such as kale, spinach, and collard greens, as well as broccoli, beets, and artichokes, can help keep the liver healthy and promote the production of healthy bile. Avoiding alcohol is essential while on antibiotics, since it increases the likelihood of liver toxicity.

10. Skip the acid suppression. Blocking stomach acid and taking an antibiotic is a recipe for microbial disaster since the lack of stomach acid leaves you vulnerable to overgrowth of pathogenic bacteria such as *C. diff* that can lead to serious infection. If you think you may require an antibiotic, try to stop any acid-suppressing drugs seventy-two hours beforehand and while taking the antibiotic to allow levels of stomach acid to return to normal.

TABLE 11–3 • Medications to Avoid

When it comes to preserving the health of your microbes, all drugs are not created equal. A five-day course of some broad-spectrum antibiotics can wipe out as much as one-third of your gut bacteria, with no guarantee that you'll ever have full regrowth, even with lots of probiotics. But antibiotics aren't the only threat. Lots of other commonly used prescription and over-the-counter medications can wreak havoc on your microbes, particularly with habitual use. It's important to know which drugs are the most problematic and to avoid them whenever possible, particularly if you've already been diagnosed with dysbiosis. An exhaustive list is beyond the scope of this book, but the list below hits the high points to be aware of in some key drug categories.

Antibiotics

- Especially broad-spectrum ones that have activity against lots of different bacteria.
- Topical creams, gels, and ointments that can cause AAD and colitis, in addition to disrupting the microbial environment on the skin.

Acid-Suppressing Drugs

- Proton pump inhibitors, histamine blockers, antacids— particularly when used for more than eight consecutive weeks.
- Note: When discontinuing proton pump inhibitors, you may experience a surge in acid production. Tapering off of the medication slowly over a few weeks can help ease the transition.

Corticosteroids

- Oral or intravenous forms are the most detrimental.
- Long-term use of inhaled steroids or steroid creams can also affect your microbiome and lead to localized fungal infections, bacterial overgrowth, or other manifestations of dysbiosis.
- Note: Oral or intravenous corticosteroids should not be abruptly discontinued—ask your doctor about a schedule for tapering them.

Birth Control Pills

- Includes pills and birth control methods like intrauterine devices (IUDs) that release hormones vaginally.
- Note: Not only used for birth control, the pills may also be prescribed for premenstrual symptoms, endometriosis, polycystic ovary syndrome (PCOS), or acne.

Hormone Replacement Therapy

- May be prescribed in pill or patch form.

Nonsteroidal Anti-inflammatory Drugs (NSAIDs)

- Includes all ibuprofen-containing drugs and aspirin.

Alternative Therapies for Common Problems

Upper Respiratory Tract/Sinus Infections

The majority of colds, flu, and sinus infections are viral, and antibiotics can actually *increase* your susceptibility to future infections (both

TABLE 11–4 · Basic Tips to Help You Protect
Your Microbiome When You're Sick

Some of the suggestions below may seem pretty intuitive. The best advice usually is—it's following it that can be tricky. These tips will help you in your efforts to break the vicious cycle of antibiotics and more illness by reminding you to give your body what it needs: rest, nourishing foods, and a little dirt.

- Stay home when you're sick.
- Strengthen your immune system by getting good sleep and cutting down on sugar.
- Rest, hydrate, and eat lots of fruits and vegetables instead of taking antibiotics for colds, flu, and other viral illnesses.
- Try to get outside and breathe fresh rather than recirculated air when you're not feeling well.
- Avoid hospitalization when possible to avoid resistant superbugs.

viral and bacterial) by depleting your body of its microbial defenses. Chronic sinusitis, one of the most common chronic ailments that affects millions of people in the United States, is itself a form of dysbiosis: sufferers have three-quarters the normal number of species present in their sinuses. Antibiotics and steroid preparations contribute to that imbalance, increasing the likelihood of future infections and making bacteria more resistant, so the severity of infections increases. Antibiotic and steroid use can also increase your risk for fungal infections—a leading but underdiagnosed cause of chronic sinusitis. Researchers at the Mayo Clinic found that a whopping 96 percent of chronic sinusitis patients—most of whom used antibiotics or steroids in the past for acute infections—had fungi in their sinus passages that were triggering an immune response and contributing to the chronic irritation and inflammation.

Before you take steroids or antibiotics, or commit to more drastic measures such as surgery, you may want to try these simple remedies for relieving your sinus symptoms:

- Stay hydrated with plenty of water, herbal teas, and broth to help thin out mucus and unclog sinus passages.
- Eliminate excess sugar from your diet to discourage the growth of fungi and other pathogenic bacteria. The Live Dirty, Eat Clean Diet is a great place to start.
- Take a robust daily probiotic with at least fifty billion colony-forming units—see Chapter 12 for specific recommendations.
- Consider trying a natural antifungal such as oregano oil (three drops in a glass of water, twice daily) if you've been on a lot of antibiotics or steroids and think you may have fungal growth.
- Use a neti pot—a container designed to rinse debris from your nasal cavity available at most pharmacies and health food stores—to help remove excess mucus, pollen, and other irritants (use distilled water rather than tap water, and add a pinch of sea salt).
- Try peppermint, eucalyptus, or rosemary oil aromatherapy. Add a few drops to a bowl of very hot water, cover your head with a towel, and lean over the bowl to allow the steam to penetrate your sinus passages.

Urinary Tract Infections

The first order of business is to make sure you really have a urinary tract infection (UTI). Bladder irritation from interstitial cystitis, or encroachment from endometriosis, fibroids, diverticulosis, or a full colon pressing on your bladder can all simulate the signs and symptoms of a UTI, including urinary urgency, frequency, burning, and pelvic pain. Many medical practices have gotten into the habit of treating first and asking questions later, and some don't even bother to send a urine specimen for analysis and culture. More than five to ten white blood cells found on urinalysis may indicate infection, but it should be confirmed with a urine culture that shows more than one hundred thousand colony-forming units (CFU) on a "clean-catch" urine specimen (i.e., obtained midstream).

Some people's urinary systems are chronically colonized with bacteria and they have positive urine cultures and abnormal urinalyses all the time. Decisions about treatment need to be personalized and made in the context of symptoms and past history. Conversely, there's debate about whether a UTI can be diagnosed despite significantly lower levels of growth on the urine culture, but that's also a specific problem that needs to be evaluated on an individual basis. Overall, the trend I've observed is overdiagnosis and treatment of symptoms in the absence of any proven infection.

Many of the patients I see with urinary symptoms have diverticulosis or constipation rather than any urinary tract pathology. Their distended colon presses on their bladder and creates pelvic discomfort that mimics a UTI. This is especially common in women because the lower part of the female colon lies deep in the pelvis adjacent to the bladder. Adding a fiber supplement to help clean out the colon usually brings relief.

Taking lots of antibiotics, even for culture-proven UTIs, can put you at risk for more infections by reducing the population of beneficial bacteria in your GI tract, allowing more undesirable species to overgrow and become more resistant and aggressive. When these pathogenic gut bacteria (usually *E. coli*) stray into the vicinity of the bladder, they can result in a UTI.

Even though this is an area rife with overdiagnosis, there are some circumstances where you don't want to allow a urinary tract infection to go undiagnosed or untreated. Fever, chills, or flank pain may indicate an upper urinary tract infection involving the kidneys (pyelonephritis), for which you should seek immediate medical care. For those with more minor symptoms, here are some ideas to help prevent UTIs and relieve symptoms:

- Hydrate, hydrate, and hydrate some more to flush your urinary system. Aim for at least eight glasses of water daily.
- Take D-mannose: one teaspoon or two grams, four times a day, for five days. D-mannose is a naturally occurring substance found in cranberries that helps prevent *E. coli* bacteria from sticking to the wall of the bladder and setting up shop. D-mannose can also be taken prophylactically; that is, to prevent infection if you're prone to UTIs.
- Empty your bladder frequently, especially after intercourse.
- Wipe front to back after bowel movements (most UTIs are caused by bacteria from the GI tract gaining entrance to the urinary tract).

Acne/Rosacea

Antibiotics are part of the problem, not the solution, if you're prone to acne and rosacea. Since these conditions are frequently a result of imbalance between naturally occurring *Propionibacterium acnes* on the skin and more troublesome *Staphylococcus* species (or, in the case of rosacea, Demodex mites), restoring beneficial microbes rather than depleting them should be the mainstay of therapy. People who've been prescribed long-term antibiotics (sometimes for decades!) for acne typically have the most challenging form of dysbiosis to treat. Antibiotics used for the skin are also very potent against gut bacteria, so the microbiome is usually quite decimated, particularly if accompanied by a dysbiosis-promoting diet high in sugar and dairy.

It's shocking that we still tell teenagers that what they eat doesn't have any effect on their skin and then subject them to years of antibiotics that can have serious effects on their health. Almost all of the patients I see in my practice with Crohn's disease and ulcerative colitis have a history of taking antibiotics for acne, and while that doesn't necessarily prove causation in those particular patients, the medical literature is full of studies that now confirm that antibiotic use, particularly in childhood, is a major risk factor for the development of these diseases.

While there are multiple other factors besides diet and antibiotics that contribute to skin problems (including genetic, environmental, and hormonal influences), in my experience, avoiding antibiotics and making significant dietary changes are part of a successful approach to getting acne and rosacea under control.

- Avoid oral and topical antibiotics to treat your acne or rosacea.
- Eliminate processed grains, sugar (including artificial sweeteners), and dairy from your diet. They influence the dominant species present on your skin and are major contributors to skin blemishes.
- Eat at least three servings of fresh leafy green vegetables such as spinach, kale, or chard daily.
- Try organic or wild-crafted (organically grown without the certification) essential oils such as tea tree or thyme. In a 2012 UK study from Leeds, tincture of thyme was found to have a greater effect on acne than a standard concentration of benzoyl peroxide—the common ingredient in most acne treatments.
- Take a robust daily probiotic with at least fifty billion colony-forming units (see Chapter 12 for specific recommendations).
- Avoid medicated acne washes, soaps, or cleansers. Use manuka honey and filtered water to wash your face (see the Oily Skin Facial Scrub and Dry Skin Facial Scrub recipes on pages 146–147), and organic jojoba oil to moisturize.
- Don't wash or cleanse your face more than once daily, as cleansing strips your face of its natural oils and can cause your skin to over-produce pore-clogging sebum.
- Take a break from makeup or give it up altogether. Even "natural" formulations can clog pores or irritate your skin. Once your skin clears up, you won't need to disguise blemishes with foundation.
- If you have rosacea, pay attention to potential dietary triggers such as sugar, alcohol, or spicy foods.
- Develop a regular meditation practice to decrease stress and help clear up acne and rosacea.

Having Your Baby the Way Nature Intended

A drug-free vaginal delivery isn't just for hippies. It's something we should all strive for, given the consequences of antibiotics and C-sections on a newborn's burgeoning microbiome. Allowing nature to take its course and not inducing labor prematurely, avoiding unnecessary medications and procedures during childbirth, and nursing as soon as possible after delivery all seem like commonsense ideas, so the fact that you need an actual document spelling it all out for your medical team tells you something about how far we've come from any notion of delivery being natural.

As I described in Chapter 7, my own childbirth experience involved uterine and external monitors, IVs, medications, surgery, and lots and lots of antibiotics. Despite being a physician—or maybe because of it—I thought all this modern medical technology was just great. I couldn't have been more wrong, and one of my biggest regrets is that I wasn't more informed about the long-term consequences of some of these interventions. It's wonderful to have medical technology and pharmaceuticals at your disposal when you need them, but for the vast majority of women giving birth, they're an unnecessary hindrance. Here's the birth plan I wish I had known about when I was pregnant. My sincerest wish is that it helps you bring a healthy baby into the world safely, replete with all the right germs necessary to have a good start.

TABLE 11–5 • Sample Pregnancy and Birth Plan/Goals

I understand that certain emergency or other medical circumstances may not allow for the accommodation of the goals listed below, but I appreciate your consideration in helping me achieve my objective of a natural childbirth.

Pregnancy Goals

- I would like to avoid antibiotics and other medications during my pregnancy unless I need to be treated for a condition that threatens my health or the health of my baby.
- As long as my baby and I are healthy and there are no medical contraindications, I would like to go at least ten to fourteen days past my due date before consideration of inducing labor.

Labor Goals

- I am trying to have as natural a birth experience as possible, with invasive procedures, tests, medications, and other interventions initiated only when medically necessary.
- I prefer not to have an IV administered unless medically necessary.
- I prefer not to have a urinary catheter placed unless medically necessary.
- Please keep the lights dim and noise to a minimum for a calm birth environment.
- I would like the opportunity to be out of bed as much as possible during labor.
- I would prefer not to undergo internal vaginal exams unless they are medically necessary.
- I would like to avoid internal fetal monitoring unless medically necessary and request that external monitoring be kept to a safe minimum.
- I prefer not to have my membranes broken unless medically necessary.
- If induction or augmentation of labor is necessary, I would like to try walking, changing positions, or nipple stimulation before being given any medications.
- I am especially interested in avoiding induction of labor with oxytocin (Pitocin).
- I will ask for pain medication only if I'm too uncomfortable to handle the pain—please don't administer it without my consent.

- I would like to utilize massage, relaxation techniques, shower, and whirlpool tub to help manage my pain.
- In the event that medication is deemed medically necessary, I would like the opportunity to discuss risks and alternatives with my obstetric team.

Delivery Goals

- I would like my baby to be placed on my chest immediately after birth with skin-to-skin contact in order to bond and nurse.
- I would like to breast-feed my baby as soon as possible after delivery.
- Please do not administer any medications to my baby, including but not limited to antibiotics, without my consent.
- Please do not use any antibacterial products, soaps, or sanitizers on my baby without my consent.
- I would prefer that any tests needed to be done to my baby be performed while he or she is on my chest.

Cesarean Section Goals

- I would like to avoid a C-section unless it is a medical necessity for my health or the health of my baby.
- I would like to be conscious during the C-section.
- Please consider allowing my baby to be wiped down immediately after the C-section with a swab of my vaginal secretions to mimic passage through the birth canal and to allow colonization with essential microbes.
- I would like to be allowed to breast-feed my baby immediately or as soon as possible after the C-section.
- I prefer to have my baby remain in the recovery room with me after the C-section.

Breast-feeding Goals

- I would like to breast-feed, so please do not offer any bottles to my baby unless medically necessary, and not without notifying me ahead of time.

- I prefer to have a private room, if available, and that my baby stay with me in the room.
- If my baby is not staying in the room with me, I would like my baby to be brought to me as frequently as necessary to satisfy his or her feeding needs.
- I would like to meet with a lactation consultant before leaving the hospital to help ensure successful breast-feeding.

It's OK to Be Sick

In order to be well, we sometimes have to be sick. We have a lot to gain by raising the bar for our own tolerance of discomfort, and dealing with minor illnesses and aches and pains without resorting to remedies that can have devastating long-term consequences. People often think: *I can't be sick, I have an important event,* or *I have a deadline at work.* But nowhere in the tried-and-true prescription of rest, hydration, and proper nourishment is there a magical fix or an instant cure that's effective and without repercussions.

For those who are truly ill, modern medicine can offer some awesome options. But for many of the complaints that we're being overtreated for, short-term pharmaceutical fixes are part of the problem, not the solution. They weaken our natural microbial defenses, rendering us more prone to illness and more dependent on drugs. By crippling our microbiome, they move us away from, rather than toward, better health. The next time you have a cold, stay in bed and drink some veggie soup instead of taking an antibiotic. Choose short-term discomfort over long-term disease. You just might find yourself healthier than ever.

CHAPTER 12

||||||||||||||||||||||||||||||||||||||||||

Bugs over Drugs: Probiotics and Other Supplements

A FIVE-DAY COURSE OF antibiotics can suppress as much as a third of your gut bacteria, and although many of these species will eventually return, the process of repopulation may take months or even years. The reality is that many of us with a damaged microbiome may never regain our full complement of essential bacteria, which is why avoidance of microbe-depleting practices is so important. In the future, we may be able to analyze our microbiome, figure out what's missing, and reliably restock it with a customized probiotic blend, but, for now, methods of repopulating our essential bacteria are still in their infancy, and much of what we know is through trial and error or anecdote.

In this chapter, I'll share what we do know, including which conditions respond best to probiotics, the limitations and risks, how to choose one, and the utility of commercially available strains. I'll also discuss a few supplements and herbal remedies that can have a beneficial effect on your microbiome. I hope this information will be helpful to you on your journey toward microbial optimization and better health.

First, a Few Definitions

Probiotics are defined by the World Health Organization as "live microorganisms which, when administered in adequate amounts, confer a health benefit on the host." Basically, they're live bacteria, usually ingested in pill, powder, or liquid form.

Prebiotics are non-digestible foods or ingredients that promote the growth of beneficial microorganisms in the intestines. In other words, they're food for your gut bacteria. Examples of prebiotics include oats, bananas, onions, garlic, leeks, asparagus, and artichokes—all of which are part of the Live Dirty, Eat Clean Diet.

Synbiotics are a combination of prebiotics and probiotics that are found primarily in fermented foods such as pickles, sauerkraut, kimchi, and kefir. In addition to being good food for gut bacteria, they also provide significant amounts of live bacteria themselves. Cabbage, for example, is high in indigestible plant fiber that can nourish gut microbes, but when fermented to sauerkraut, it also provides *Lactobacillus* species.

How Do Probiotics Improve Health?

Probiotics have been used for medicinal purposes for centuries. The Romans advocated the use of fermented raw milk as an antidote for gastrointestinal infections, and in the early 1900s, Russian scientist Élie Metchnikoff promoted the use of probiotics after noticing that Bulgarians who consumed lots of fermented products seemed to live longer. We still don't know all the ways that probiotics can improve human health, but some of the mechanisms include:

- Suppression of pathogens
- Stimulation of the immune system
- Reduction of inflammation
- Destruction of toxins

- Production of essential vitamins
- Improvement of the integrity of the gut lining/epithelial barrier

Indications for Taking a Probiotic

Popping a probiotic has become as popular as taking vitamins—and, for many people, just as ineffectual. There's a tremendous amount of money to be made by convincing everyone that they're better off with a probiotic than without one. Before you commit, it's important to know whether there's any data to suggest that a probiotic can help the condition you're trying to treat, or whether your resources would be better spent pursuing more promising treatment options. For some disorders, such as antibiotic-associated diarrhea (AAD), it's intuitive that replacing gut bacteria would be helpful. But more and more data are pointing to a role for probiotics in a number of diverse and seemingly unrelated conditions, from anxiety and depression to high cholesterol and fatigue.

A study published in the journal *Proceedings of the National Academy of Sciences* suggested that probiotic bacteria might have the potential to change brain neurochemistry and treat anxiety and depression-related disorders, which is consistent with existing data showing that anxiety can actually be induced in germ-free mice by transferring gut bacteria from anxious mice. Research presented at the American Heart Association meeting in 2012 described a *Lactobacillus* strain that, when administered, resulted in a reduction of blood levels of LDL or "bad" cholesterol, and other *Lactobacillus* strains have been found to protect against infection with *Listeria*. Scientists at University College Cork, Ireland, reported that *Bifidobacterium*, which is known to be helpful for irritable bowel syndrome, may also have benefits for patients with psoriasis and chronic fatigue syndrome.

There still isn't enough data to recommend the routine use of probiotics for all of these disorders, but in the near future we may see more opportunities for disease intervention utilizing specific strains of bacteria.

The following tables list conditions where there's scientific evidence that probiotics are helpful, and some conditions for which there might not be many clinical studies but enough anecdotal evidence to suggest that probiotics may be of benefit.

TABLE 12–1 • Conditions That Are Helped by Probiotics

- Acne
- Antibiotic-associated diarrhea (AAD)
- Bacterial vaginosis (BV)
- *Clostridium difficile (C. diff)*
- Dysbiosis
- Infectious diarrhea
- Inflammatory bowel disease (IBD)
- Irritable bowel syndrome (IBS)
- Leaky gut
- Sinus infections
- Traveler's diarrhea
- Urinary tract infections (UTIs)
- Yeast infections

TABLE 12–2 • Conditions That *May* Be Helped by Probiotics

- Allergies
- Anxiety/depression
- Autism
- Autoimmune diseases
- Chronic fatigue syndrome
- Heart disease
- Obesity

Limitations and Risks of Taking Probiotics

Probiotics have a long safety record, but, as with any therapeutic modality, there can be risk involved. Formulations can become contaminated with harmful strains, and in someone who has a compromised immune system, even benign bacteria can be a hazard. Transfer of harmful genes and overstimulation of the immune system are rare but are among the more serious potential side effects. We don't know much about the effects of probiotics in the elderly or in very young children, so these are areas where caution should be exercised. For the average person, side effects are usually mild and include gas, bloating, nausea, and occasionally diarrhea. When I prescribe a robust probiotic containing large amounts of bacteria, I'll usually tell my patients to start with a quarter dose or half dose and increase gradually to the full amount over three to four weeks so that their body has time to get used to it.

There are very few randomized placebo controlled trials (the gold standard for scientific investigation) that have studied the benefits of probiotics, so we rely heavily on a trial-and-error approach and anecdotal results. Cause and effect can be difficult to discern because many people are predisposed to believe that the probiotic they're taking is helpful, which can bias their opinion about whether it's truly beneficial. People also tend to modify their diet when they start a probiotic, so it can be hard to tell which intervention is responsible for any improvement.

More research is definitely needed to understand how the microbiome is affected by factors such as age, genetics, the environment, and diet, and, consequently, which species may help restore a damaged microbiome at various stages of life or for distinct diseases. Different types of bacteria perform different functions in the body, and species that are beneficial at a young age might actually be harmful in an older person. For example, *Helicobacter pylori* seems to have a protective effect in childhood but has been associated with ulcers and even cancer later in life, so the role of various microbes may change as we age, making it even more challenging to figure out which ones we should be taking.

One of the biggest obstacles to creating a beneficial probiotic may be the fact that many of the microbial species within the gastrointestinal (GI) tract have not yet been discovered. For the ones we do know about, not all can be successfully cultured and grown outside of the body, and kept alive on the shelf in a capsule or powder. We can't replace bacteria that we can't cultivate. Finally, even those of us who are enthusiastic about probiotics and recommend them for a wide range of conditions have to acknowledge that the marketplace is rife with overselling of their potential benefits. Even though they're mostly innocuous, probiotics are still a type of medicine, and they should be held to the same reasonable standards as other therapeutic interventions: they should improve your health without doing you harm.

How Long Before You See Results?

The answer to this question is: I don't know. It depends on the condition you're treating, how damaged your microbiome is, your diet, your overall health, and the potency of the probiotic you're using. The probiotic I use most frequently in my practice (besides my own Gutbliss brand) is a high-dose formulation called VSL#3, which is considered a medical food for the treatment of inflammatory bowel disease (IBD). It's available in capsules and a higher-strength powder, as well as in a double-strength prescription form containing nine hundred billion colony-forming units (CFU) of various strains of *Bifidobacteria*, *Lactobacillus*, and *Streptococcus*. Most of my patients with dysbiosis notice improvement within approximately sixty days, although the range can be a few weeks to several months.

In general, the longer you've been on antibiotics, the longer it takes for probiotics to take effect. For some people who are trying to remediate years of chronic antibiotic use, it can take several months or even a year for them to see meaningful results. Since probiotics don't necessarily colonize the intestine and a lot of the bacteria simply pass through and are excreted, you may need to take probiotics indefinitely to experience continued benefits.

Taking combinations of different probiotic formulations that aren't designed to work together isn't usually a good idea. More is not necessarily merrier when it comes to probiotics, since different strains may compete with each other or interact negatively.

Unfortunately, some people who take probiotics don't get better, either because there's too much microbial or cellular damage, or because dysbiosis isn't really the cause of their problem—something worth considering if you've been taking a probiotic for a long time and aren't seeing results. Like any medical intervention, appropriate supervision by a health care professional is recommended.

How to Choose a Probiotic

Important factors to consider when choosing a probiotic include whether it contains sufficient numbers of live bacteria, as well as the right strains to confer a health benefit for the condition you're trying to treat (not whether it helped your neighbor or your yoga instructor, who may have had a completely different problem than you do). Although there's no one-size-fits-all version when it comes to probiotics, here's some general advice for choosing a probiotic:

- Probiotics on the market may contain from one billion to nine hundred billion CFU. Pick one with at least fifty billion CFU of the two most important groups of probiotic bacteria: *Lactobacilli* and *Bifidobacteria*.
- Make sure the product contains multiple compatible strains of bacteria designed to work together, since different strains have different

functions and no one strain can provide all the benefits. Most robust probiotics contain at least seven different strains.

- Choose a probiotic with enteric coating to protect the bacteria from being destroyed by stomach acid.
- Make sure the product has a good safety record with regard to human use. Check the Internet to see whether any clinical trials or other scientific studies have been done to assess side effects, or whether the manufacturer provides any safety information.
- Investigate whether it has activity against pathogenic bacteria. Check the Internet to see whether any clinical trials or other scientific studies have been done to assess efficacy in people with active infections, or whether the manufacturer provides any information on activity against pathogens.
- Check to see what the shelf life is, whether the product needs to be refrigerated, and whether it's stable under normal storage conditions.
- The manufacturer should guarantee that the product was tested and certify that it contains the amount of live bacteria stated on the label. This should be on the package label or insert.
- There are several companies that claim to independently test health products like probiotics for purity and strength to help consumers identify the best-quality ones, but many of them receive grants and funding from the probiotic manufacturers whose products they endorse, so the information is not always unbiased. When you're doing your research, look for data unencumbered by a financial relationship.

TABLE 12–3 • Common Probiotic Strains

- *Lactobacillus acidophilus* ferments sugars into lactic acid and produces amylase, which helps digest carbohydrates. It's one of the most popular probiotics and is used commercially in many dairy products. It's highly resistant to stomach acid and adheres well to intestinal cells, helping to prevent the proliferation of opportunistic species (essentially taking up all the bar stools so bad bacteria can't get a drink). It's especially helpful for restoring the natural flora in bacterial vaginosis.
- *Lactobacillus casei* is found in the mouth and intestines, and also in fermented vegetables, milk, and meat. It seems to inhibit the growth of *Helicobacter pylori* and has shown efficacy in combination with other strains in alleviating gastrointestinal (GI) conditions such as antibiotic-associated and infectious diarrhea. *L. casei* can complement the proliferation of *L. acidophilus* and can also be used in the fermentation of beans to reduce gas-producing, poorly digested carbohydrates.
- *Lactobacillus rhamnosus* is very hardy and resistant to stomach acid and bile. It's present in the mouth and in the GI tract, and also in the vagina and urinary tract of women, where it can prevent pathogens from gaining a foothold. *L. rhamnosus* has been used successfully to treat diarrhea caused by rotavirus, as well as some forms of atopic dermatitis (AD). Despite its many uses as a probiotic, it's been associated with infection in people with a weakened immune system.
- *Lactobacillus salivarius* suppresses pathogenic bacteria and reduces gas in people with irritable bowel syndrome (IBS). It may also be helpful in cases of pancreatitis by suppressing harmful bacteria in the GI tract that can contaminate the pancreas.
- *Streptococcus thermophilus* is found in fermented milk products such as yogurt and can help digest lactose in the intestines.
- *Bifidobacterium bifidum* is part of the normal flora of the large intestine and, like *Lactobacillus acidophilus*, is also one of the most

common probiotics. It helps break down and absorb simple sugars and has been shown to increase immune function by decreasing severity of symptoms and length of illness from the common cold. It's present in the vagina and helpful for treating candida and other forms of yeast overgrowth.

- *Bifidobacterium longum* is one of the founding species in infants, and it thrives in the low-oxygen environment of the colon. It helps prevent the growth of pathogens by producing lactic acid, and can also improve lactose tolerance, prevent diarrhea, and ameliorate allergies. *B. longum* may play a role in cancer prevention through alteration of the pH of the colon, and it reduces the risk for atherosclerosis and stroke through scavenging free radicals. It's a common addition to food products because of its beneficial effects.

- *Bifidobacterium lactis* is also known as *B. animalis*. Its beneficial effects on abdominal discomfort and bloating in people with constipation-predominant IBS are well described, and in clinical trials it was shown to protect intestinal cells from damage by gluten in people with celiac disease. It's commonly used in dairy products.

Supplements

Almost every supplement these days claims to be good for your microbiome or to boost your immune system in some way. But getting your nutrients from food instead of through a supplement is always preferable because you get the entire spectrum of health-promoting ingredients when you eat the whole food, instead of just one isolated constituent that's often accompanied by undesirable fillers and binders. Green powders that claim to be the equivalent of eating vegetables are a particular pet peeve of mine, since most vegetables start to wilt and lose their nutrient value shortly after harvesting. The idea that important nutrients in these foods can still be active years after they're extracted just isn't plausible—or proven.

Fructooligosaccharides (FOS) are poorly digestible carbohydrates that occur naturally in foods high in inulin, such as onions, chicory, garlic, asparagus, bananas, and artichokes. They have a prebiotic effect that's been well documented in studies using both the actual foods and inulin supplementation. Psyllium husk is another form of plant fiber with prebiotic effects that also helps with symptoms of dysbiosis by bulking the stool and moving the products of digestion through in a timely fashion, preventing stasis (constipation) and uncomfortable gas. I still recommend eating large amounts of high-fiber foods, but taking a few grams of inulin or psyllium husk powder as well can be a good idea to boost your fiber intake.

My fear is always that patients will take supplements in lieu of eating the right foods, which won't get them very far in terms of tangible health benefits. For these reasons, I'm generally not a fan of supplements and advocate a nutrient-dense diet over shelf-stable pills and powders. That said, there are a few supplements that can be helpful in the treatment of dysbiosis when used in conjunction with a diet rich in indigestible plant fiber. Some work by inhibiting unhealthy bacteria, while others boost levels of beneficial bacteria or have proven antiparasitic, antifungal, or antiviral effects. Here are some you should know about:

TABLE 12–4 • Supplements That Are Useful in Treating Dysbiosis

- **Berberine**—active against *Candida albicans* and *Staphylococcus aureus*
- **Enteric-coated peppermint oil**—helpful in small intestinal bacterial overgrowth (SIBO) and IBS
- **Garlic**—active against bacteria, fungi, viruses, and parasites

- **Glutamine**—helpful for repairing the lining of the gut in dysbiosis and leaky gut
- **Grapefruit seed extract**—has antimicrobial and antifungal activity
- **Inulin**—fermentable fiber with prebiotic properties that increases growth of beneficial bacteria
- **Olive leaf extract**—has anti-inflammatory and antibacterial effects
- **Oregano oil**—good for nail fungus and sinus infections; also has antiparasitic effects
- **Psyllium husk**—plant-based fiber with prebiotic and stool-bulking properties
- **Tea tree oil**—has natural antifungal properties
- **Turmeric/curcumin**—has anti-inflammatory properties and boosts immune function
- **Wormwood**—antiparasitic agent, but has some risks, so should be medically supervised
- **Zinc**—enhances barrier function of the gut

You Can't Hack Your Microbiome

When it comes to your microbiome, an ounce of prevention is definitely worth a pound of cure: it's better to avoid depleting your microbes in the first place than to try to replace them with significantly less robust store-bought versions. It took an entire lifetime to amass the trillions of bacteria that call your gut home, but just one course of antibiotics can wreak serious havoc on them, especially when accompanied by a standard Western diet high in fat and sugar. There's no magic wand for quickly and reliably undoing that damage, although, over time, a carefully chosen probiotic can help to restore depleted species. Probiotics aren't a panacea, but for those suffering from dysbiosis and other modern plagues for which microbial discord may be the root cause, they represent a glimmer of real hope for improved health.

CHAPTER 13

||||||||||||||||||||||||||||||||||||||||||||

Everything You Wanted to Know About Stool Transplants but Were Afraid to Ask

WHILE I WAS writing this book, I got a call from a friend who'd undergone eight weeks of antibiotic therapy for Lyme disease and wanted to know whether a stool transplant might be in order to restore his microbiome. Other than some gas, a fouler-than-usual odor to his stools, and a mild but itchy rash on his back, he was feeling close to his usual baseline. He hadn't developed *C. diff* from the antibiotics and had no history of inflammatory bowel disease (IBD) or other autoimmune conditions.

My advice to him was that fecal microbiota transplant (FMT)—a fancy name for a not-so-fancy procedure—was probably not a good idea. His microbiome had definitely taken a hit after all those antibiotics, but there wasn't a clear indication for treatment, and transplanting stool from someone else—even a close someone like his girlfriend—came with risks, including transferring harmful microbes along with the good ones. I explained that since he was basically healthy and hadn't taken a lot of antibiotics prior to being treated for Lyme disease, his microbiome would likely recover to an acceptable baseline over time. If he developed more worrisome signs and symptoms down the road, such as persistent diarrhea, or features of Crohn's disease or ulcer-ative colitis, it would be worth reconsidering the utility of a stool transplant, but for now I recommended that he take several months of a robust probiotic, increase his dietary fiber, and cut down on sugary, starchy food and alcohol. (I also told him that he should have pressed his doctor about whether a shorter course of treatment for the Lyme disease was possible.)

Straight to the Source

FMT may seem like a drastic way to rehab your microbiome, but there's lots of precedence for going straight to the source when it comes to ac-quiring gut bacteria. Farmers have long known that digestive illnesses in cows can be successfully treated by feeding the sick cow the intesti-nal contents that have been sucked out of a healthy cow's stomach. Coprophagia, or eating stool, is common in the animal kingdom: baby elephants, pandas, koalas, and hippos eat the feces of their mother or other adults in their herd in order to acquire vital gut bacteria required for digestion. Consumption of fresh camel feces has been observed among certain tribes, including the Bedouin, as a highly effective treat-ment for infectious diarrhea. And in medieval times it was not uncom-mon for physicians to taste their patient's stool to aid in diagnosis—a practice I'm in no hurry to resurrect.

Indications for FMT

We've come a long way—from being grossed out by our own stool to contemplating consuming other people's. As a gastroenterologist who believes wholeheartedly in the hygiene hypothesis and the importance of rewilding, FMT represents a fascinating and logical way to tackle severe microbial discord by increasing rather than decreasing our bac-terial load. There's still a lot we don't know about FMT—including which conditions benefit the most; who makes an ideal donor; how many transplants we need to do; whether ingestible capsules work as well as enemas—but the answers are coming at breakneck speed as clinicians, scientists, and patients embrace and explore the amazing world of stool.

Clostridium difficile

FMT is now considered the most effective therapy for refractory *Clostridium difficile* (*C. diff*) infection in people who have not been helped by antibiotic therapy. With a response rate of over 90 percent, FMT may soon become first-line therapy for *C. diff*, even before treatment with antibiotics. The response to FMT is rapid for *C. diff*—a few days in most cases and just hours in some. People with IBD are at increased risk for *C. diff*, so co-infection is common and needs to be excluded in anyone who has recently taken antibiotics and is experiencing a flare-up of IBD symptoms. Most clinical trials, and my own experience at Georgetown Hospital with my colleague Mark Mattar, MD, indicate that one FMT is sufficient to treat *C. diff* in most people, but in those with IBD, additional treatments are often necessary.

Inflammatory Bowel Disease

More and more evidence points to the role of microbial imbalance and reduced microbial diversity in the pathogenesis of IBD. Early studies utilizing FMT to treat ulcerative colitis show amelioration of symptoms as well as the possibility of sustained remission and even cure. Large clinical trials demonstrate improvement in symptoms and cessation of medications in 76 percent of patients and remission in 63 percent.

Unlike *C. diff*, where the response is swift, with ulcerative colitis it takes longer for symptoms to improve after FMT, and the improvement may increase over time as the microbiome gradually shifts toward normalcy. FMT also works for Crohn's disease, although the results from clinical trials have not been as impressive as those for ulcerative colitis, and achieving lasting remission is more elusive.

Irritable Bowel Syndrome

Although there's evidence to suggest efficacy of FMT in people with IBS, especially the diarrhea-predominant subtype, the results have not been as dramatic as those for *C. diff.* Post-infectious IBS that develops after a bout of dysentery (a.k.a. traveler's diarrhea) or IBS in someone with a history of lots of antibiotic use may have features that predict a favorable response to FMT. In a small study at Montefiore Medical Center in New York City, FMT resolved or improved symptoms in 70 percent of patients with refractory IBS and resulted in improved quality of life in almost half. Careful exclusion of other etiologies of IBS that may not be microbially based is a must before consideration of FMT.

Obesity, Diabetes, and Metabolic Syndrome

Other conditions associated with a disordered microbiome are natural candidates for FMT therapy, but we still need large-scale clinical trials that can tell us how effective FMT really is for these conditions. Pilot studies investigating the effects of transferring stool from lean donors to obese recipients showed improved insulin sensitivity and increased production of beneficial short-chain fatty acids (SCFAs), although most studies were too short to assess meaningful changes in weight. FMT by itself is probably not helpful for obesity, diabetes, or metabolic syndrome without a significant dietary change—which for some people may be all they need in order to effect meaningful changes in their microbiome.

TABLE 13-1 • Indications for FMT

The following conditions all have clinical data to support the use of FMT, although FMT is not first-line therapy for any of them and should only be considered after standard treatments, including significant dietary modification and probiotics, have proved ineffective.

- *Clostridium difficile* (*C. diff*)
- Crohn's disease
- Infectious diarrhea
- Irritable bowel syndrome (IBS)
- Pouchitis (after colectomy for ulcerative colitis)
- Severe antibiotic-associated diarrhea (AAD)
- Ulcerative colitis

TABLE 13-2 • Potential Indications for FMT

While there is anecdotal evidence to support the use of FMT in the management of these disorders, we're still waiting for more extensive clinical trials to document a clear benefit.

- Autism
- Autoimmune disorders
- Diabetes
- Leaky gut
- Metabolic syndrome
- Obesity
- Small intestinal bacterial overgrowth (SIBO)

How Quickly Will You Notice a Change?

For the best-studied indication—refractory *Clostridium difficile* (*C. diff*)—more than 50 percent of patients experience relief of symptoms within three days, although the time frame ranges from within hours after the transplant to about six days. For chronic autoimmune conditions, there's typically much more microbial discord than there is with an acute event like *C. diff*, so the response time tends to be much longer. In those cases, it can be several weeks before seeing any meaningful improvement, although there may be some glimmers of amelioration before then. It's hard to say what's a reasonable amount of time to wait before deciding that FMT isn't working for you, because there are no clinical guidelines to help make those determinations, but if after ten to twelve transplants within two months there's really no improvement, it's probably time to move on.

How Often Does FMT Need to Be Done?

Frequency of FMT really depends on the indication. Studies show that the majority of people with *C. diff* respond to just one FMT. And when researchers compared post-transplant *C. diff* patients with healthy individuals in a control group, they found that both groups had similar bacterial environments, suggesting that even one transplant was able to restore a diverse community of healthy gut bacteria. This makes sense for a self-limited infectious event like *C. diff* in an otherwise healthy person, but, as mentioned earlier, long-standing dysbiosis is much more challenging to treat.

For chronic autoimmune illnesses such as Crohn's and ulcerative colitis, you may need to do an initial series of daily FMT for one to two weeks, followed by a regimen of one to three times a week indefinitely, or at least for several months. Remember that most of the bacteria you're transplanting don't take up residence in the colon—they just pass through—although they may reproduce while in your digestive tract. So although some people are able to achieve lasting changes in their microbial composition and then stop treatment, for most autoimmune diseases, FMT represents an ongoing form of therapy that needs to be administered regularly. The good news is that for some patients with IBD, the effects of FMT continue to improve over time as the microbial changes slowly take root.

Anonymous Donors, Stool Banks, and Synthetic Stool

If you're contemplating FMT, finding an appropriate donor may be your biggest challenge. It can be awkward having to ask someone whether they've used recreational drugs or had a sexually transmitted disease (STD), and then requiring them to undergo the extensive testing involved in donor screening. Seeking out an anonymous donor bypasses the challenge of finding a suitable donor among family members or friends, and also avoids the problem of shared genetic and environmental risks, which is helpful if you have a strong family history of autoimmune disease or cancer.

Commercially available screened frozen samples from "stool banks" are now being used by some hospitals, since they eliminate the need to prepare material from new donors for each transplant. Emory University Medical School has used residents from the pathology department as regular donors—perhaps the ultimate gift of healing to their patients undergoing FMT.

Researchers at Queen's University in Ontario, Canada, created a synthetic stool mixture of thirty-three different types of intestinal bacteria called RePOOPulate by culturing stool from a healthy person. They used it to successfully clear *C. diff* infection in two patients and documented that the RePOOPulate mixture made up 25 percent of the gut bacterial population in the recipients several months after the transplant. A synthetic mixture allows researchers to control which bacteria are included and reduces the possibility of harmful bacteria or viruses being transferred. Custom brews containing different species depending on the indication may be next, although the fact that not all gut bacteria can be cultured and grown is still a major limitation, as is the possibility of contamination.

In the future we may be able to culture small amounts of good bacteria from our own guts, incubate and grow them outside of the digestive tract into larger colonies without competition from pathogenic strains, and then transplant them back, sidestepping any awkward donor issues.

Modes of Administration

In the early days of FMT, the transplanted stool was administered primarily via colonoscopy, which involves a flexible tube with a light on the end that's inserted into the rectum and advanced up through the colon. Colonoscopy allows for good placement of the specimen in the colon, but it requires a bowel cleanse prep beforehand and sedation, and it comes with a much higher price tag than a do-it-yourself enema at home. In some situations where we're trying to exclude other conditions, like new-onset ulcerative colitis, or when we need to evaluate the colon for evidence of active inflammation, it may make sense to do FMT via colonoscopy.

FMT has also been done via upper endoscopy, where a smaller version of the colonoscope is inserted through the mouth and down into the stomach and small intestine. Ideally, specimens placed this way should be deposited deep in the small intestine, so the bacteria aren't destroyed by stomach acid. Upper endoscopy, too, involves sedation and has to be performed in a hospital, endoscopy suite, or doctor's office.

Some centers perform FMT by inserting a thin rubber tube, called a nasogastric tube (NGT), through the nose while the patient is awake and threading it down into the stomach. The stool specimen can then be squirted down through the tube into the stomach using a large syringe attached to the nasal end of the tube.

Several studies have shown success treating *C. diff* using ingestible stool capsules with a gel coating that dissolves and releases bacteria lower down in the intestines. It's less messy than a stool enema, but it requires swallowing a few dozen capsules.

Techniques like upper endoscopy, NGT, and stool capsules can be more convenient than introducing the stool from below, but they carry the theoretical risk that some of the bacteria will take up residence in the small intestine before getting to the colon, potentially leading to small intestinal bacterial overgrowth (SIBO). DIY stool transplants through enemas are possible if you are armed with good instructions and a consultation with your doctor. I'll describe at-home stool transplants in detail later in this chapter.

Donor Selection and Screening

In the future, we may be able to figure out which specific microbial profile, or enterotype, is best suited for which disease, and ultimately match the donor with the indication. For example, we know that children from Burkina Faso have a type 2 enterotype where *Prevotella* makes up 53 percent of the gut bacteria, while age-matched European children have a type 1 enterotype with no *Prevotella* but lots of *Bacteroides*, reflecting a Western diet with less fiber. We don't yet know if geographical adaptations mean that you're better off with the healthiest version of stool from your neck of the woods, or if a donor from another continent with an entirely different enterotype would be a better fix for your problem.

Given the principles of the hygiene hypothesis and the super-sanitized approach of more developed countries, donors from indigenous societies with more biodiverse lifestyles have a lot of appeal, assuming infectious possibilities can be reliably excluded. Just as with organ transplants, the success of FMT is ultimately based on two things: the health of the recipient and the quality of the transplanted stool. Here are a few things to keep in mind if you're contemplating a fecal transplant:

- The preferred donor should be an intimate longtime partner of the recipient, first-degree relative, or close family friend. It's important to know your donor well, including habits and past medical history, family medical history, what illnesses the donor may have been exposed to in the past, and lifestyle factors such as recreational drug use and sexually transmitted diseases. If there is a strong family history of autoimmune illnesses or cancer, a first-degree relative may not be ideal.
- Choose a donor with microbe-friendly lifestyle habits that include a healthy whole-foods diet with minimal processed foods, no smoking, regular exercise, low levels of stress, and minimal exposure to prescription drugs. Of course, the fewer antibiotics they've taken, the better (see below for antibiotic exclusion criteria).
- Ideally, donors should be over the age of eighteen to be able to give informed consent, although children can serve as donors as long as both parental consent and child agreement to serve as a donor are established.

TABLE 13-3 • Donor Exclusion Criteria

- Antibiotic treatment in the twelve months preceding donation
- History of chronic gastrointestinal (GI) illnesses, including inflammatory bowel disease (IBD), irritable bowel syndrome (IBS), celiac disease, GI malignancies, or major GI surgical procedures
- Autoimmune or allergic illnesses or currently taking immune-modulating therapy

- Fibromyalgia, chronic fatigue syndrome, or neurologic disorders such as Parkinson's disease
- Metabolic syndrome, obesity (BMI of >30), or moderate-to-severe malnutrition
- History of malignant illnesses or ongoing chemotherapy

TABLE 13-4 • Donor Testing (To Be Performed Within Four Weeks Prior to Donation)

- Hepatitis A (HAV-IgM, hepatitis A IgM antibody) blood test
- Hepatitis B (HBsAg, hepatitis B surface antigen) blood test
- Hepatitis C (anti-HCV-Ab, anti-HCV antibody test) blood test
- HIV (HIV EIA, enzyme immunoassay) blood test
- Syphilis (RPR, rapid plasma reagin) blood test
- *Clostridium difficile* stool test
- Stool culture (enteric pathogens)
- Ova and parasites stool test, if history is suggestive or if donor has traveled overseas in the past twelve months

Risks of FMT

The medical community first learned about hepatitis C virus (HCV) in the 1970s, but it wasn't until 1990 that widespread screening of blood donors was instituted, and by then, hundreds of thousands of people in the United States were already infected from tainted blood transfusions or poorly sterilized medical equipment. Although HCV isn't transmitted in stool (hepatitis A is), it serves as a reminder that there can be common but undiscovered infections that are highly contagious, and it may turn out that some of them are transmissible via stool.

Along with helpful microbes, FMT also transfers fungi, viruses,

TABLE 13–5 • Diseases and Organisms That Can Be Spread Through Stool

- Ascariasis
- Cholera
- *Clostridium difficile* (*C. diff*)
- Cryptosporidiosis
- *Entameba histolytica*
- Enteroviruses
- *Escherichia coli*
- Giardiasis
- Hepatitis A
- Hepatitis E
- Norovirus
- Poliomyelitis
- Rotavirus
- Shigella
- Tapeworms
- Typhoid fever
- *Vibrio parahaemolyticus*

bacteriophages (viruses that replicate within bacteria), and potentially harmful strains of bacteria. There's no way to selectively acquire only the helpful ones, or to be sure that harmful species may not be present. There's a lot we can test for (see Table 13–4), but there are still many organisms that haven't yet been cultivated and classified, and we don't know what effects they may ultimately have in another host.

Some microbes when present in large numbers may increase the risk for serious illnesses, such as colon cancer, or transfer harmful genes to our own native bacteria. So there is clearly risk associated with FMT, which is why an intimate, longtime partner with whom you've already swapped body fluids is the ideal donor, assuming he or she meets the inclusion and exclusion criteria.

Because this is a field that's still in its infancy, we really don't know what the long-term positive and negative effects of FMT are, but if the past few years are any indication, we'll have that information very soon as clinical trials, as well as anecdotal experience with FMT, continue to accumulate rapidly.

How to Perform FMT

There are lots of ways to perform a fecal transplant, and if FMT is going to become a regular part of your life, you'll undoubtedly figure out how best to modify things to suit your needs. I highly recommend doing this in consultation with an experienced physician who can help you determine if you're a good candidate, arrange donor screening, assist in evaluating the efficacy of the transplant, lay out a plan for the timing of future treatments, and be available to troubleshoot any issues that may arise. Here are some detailed instructions that may help:

Supplies
- Bottle of 0.9 percent sodium chloride (saline) solution
- Measuring cup
- Funnel
- Metal strainer with medium-size holes
- Dedicated basic blender (not high-speed)
- Plastic spoon
- Disposable saline enema bag
- Distilled water
- Toilet hat (for stool specimen collection, available at medical supply pharmacy)
- Plastic shower curtain
- Lubricant
- Cushion that you don't mind getting dirty
- Timer
- Reading material (optional)

Tip: get a friend (or perhaps the stool donor) to help the first time.

The Day Before
- Have a light or liquid lunch and dinner the day before so your colon won't be too full when you do the enema the next day.

- I don't recommend cleaning out your colon with an enema or laxative, or taking antibiotics beforehand, as some practitioners do.

Obtaining the Donor Stool

- The donor should raise the toilet seat, place the toilet hat under the seat toward the rear of the bowl, and lower the seat to hold the hat in place. The hat will collect the donor's stool from a bowel movement.
- Ideally, you should use the stool sample within two hours of obtaining it, since gut bacteria have a very short life span.
- If your donor has hard stool, he or she may want to consider taking a daily tablespoon of ground psyllium husk dissolved in a large glass of water, or increasing water and indigestible fiber consumption for a few weeks before the transplant to soften stool.

Preparing the Donor Stool

- Empty the entire stool sample from the toilet hat into the blender, using the plastic spoon to help if needed. Add a few ounces of 0.9 percent sodium chloride (saline) solution. Note: add the saline in incrementally if you're not sure how much to use, so you don't end up making the mixture too liquid. If the sample is too thick, it may clog the nozzle of the enema bag; if it's too watery, it will be harder to retain it in your colon after transfer. If the stool is too liquid, you can thicken it with some psyllium husk.
- Give the mixture three or four quick pulses to obtain a thick, smoothie-like consistency. Blending can introduce air into the sample and generate heat, both of which are detrimental to gut bacteria, so avoid overblending.
- Pour the prepared stool through the strainer into the measuring cup, using the plastic spoon to break up any lumps. This step is optional if the stool doesn't appear to have many lumps in it.
- Dump out the saline in the enema bag and rinse it with distilled water. Some enemas contain other ingredients besides saline, so it's best not to use the saline that comes with the enema bag.

- Make sure that the nozzle on the enema bag is in the closed position. Then, using the funnel, transfer the stool from the measuring cup into the enema bag.

Performing the Stool Transplant

- The best location for performing the transfer is in the bathtub or on the bathroom floor. Especially the first few times, it's a good idea to lie on top of a disposable plastic shower curtain, since things may get a little messy.
- It may be helpful to hang the enema bag on a hook a few inches above the height of your buttocks, so that gravity will help the contents run into your colon.
- Apply a little lubricant to your rectum.
- Lie on your left side and elevate your left hip and buttocks on a cushion.
- Raising your right leg slightly to allow passage, gently insert the enema nozzle into your rectum, and open the nozzle switch. The nozzle should glide easily into your rectum, especially if you relax with a few deep breaths. If you feel resistance, it may not be inserted correctly. Inserting a finger into your rectum ahead of time when you apply the lubricant may help with insertion of the nozzle.
- You should feel a slight fullness as the stool flows into your rectum, and some mild discomfort is normal, but if you have pain you should stop and remove the enema bag.
- Once the stool is flowing, tighten your buttocks to try and hold things in. If you feel like the stool is starting to leak out, you may be at capacity and need to close the nozzle. You can wait ten or fifteen minutes and then try to add a bit more in.
- After you've finished infusing the stool, close the nozzle and remove the enema bag.
- Spend fifteen minutes in each of these positions: first, lie on your left side; then lie on your stomach with the cushion underneath your hips to elevate your buttocks; then lie on your back; then lie

on your right side. All of this time should total one hour. This is where it's helpful to have the timer and some reading material (I highly recommend my book *Gutbliss* if you haven't read it!).

- Ideally, you should try to retain the stool transplant for at least four to six hours. It's a good idea to do the process at bedtime and keep the stool in overnight while you're lying down, although you may need to reinforce things with a sanitary pad, plastic undergarments, and a large towel or disposable plastic sheet.

- The first time is always the trickiest. After a few transplants you'll get the hang of it and figure out any adjustments you need to make.

The Next Frontier

One of my roles as a gastroenterologist is to educate people about what goes into their digestive tract and what comes out of it, so I spend a lot of time talking about food and stool. I encourage my patients—and my family members—to evaluate things from both ends, and that often means taking a closer-than-comfortable look at what's in the toilet bowl. Most of us have an aversion to stool stemming from early childhood when we're discouraged from using "potty words," passing gas, or making any references to our "poo." Bowel movements are viewed as something dirty and furtive, best flushed away quickly and not discussed in polite company, despite the fact that every human being on the planet has them on a regular, if not daily, basis.

So you can only imagine my joy when stories about stool started turning up on the front page of the *New York Times* and the *Wall Street Journal*, and everyone—from my most demure patients to my daughter's elementary school teachers—suddenly wanted to talk about fecal transplants. The fact that they work brilliantly for indications such as *C. diff* makes it all the sweeter, but just the idea that people are having these conversations, seeing stool in a whole new light, and gaining a better understanding of how their bodies work is cause for celebration.

Fecal transplants, which I like to think of as the ultimate probiotic, represent a paradigm shift in medicine—from too clean to not dirty enough. They're a great example of the importance and benefits of rewilding and of approaching illness from the perspective of how we can increase rather than decrease our microbial load. FMT may well be the poster child for the Live Dirty lifestyle—it doesn't get much dirtier than incorporating someone else's stool into your body—and the results speak for themselves.

part 4

———————

RECIPES

CHAPTER 14

|||||||||||||||||||||||||||||||||||||||||||

Microbiome Solution Recipes
All Recipes by Elise Museles of Kale & Chocolate

Sweet Potato & Kale Breakfast Hash

If you like savory morning meals but crave just a little sweetness, then you'll love this combination of kale and sweet potatoes with green apple thrown into the mix. Filled with veggies, fiber, and good complex carbs, this powerhouse breakfast is an energizing way to start the day. Top it with an egg if you prefer more protein, or sprinkle with pumpkin seeds for a vegan option.

*SERVES 2

Ingredients

- 1 tablespoon coconut oil
- 1 medium-large sweet potato, peeled and cut into ¼-inch cubes
- ½ small red onion, finely chopped
- 1 small Granny Smith apple, peeled and cut into ½-inch cubes
- 1 clove garlic, finely chopped
- ¼ teaspoon red pepper flakes

1 bunch dinosaur kale, stalks removed and sliced into thin ribbons

1 to 2 teaspoons olive oil

Sea salt to taste

1 tablespoon chopped fresh rosemary (or 1 teaspoon dried)

Method

✳ PLACE THE COCONUT OIL in a medium skillet and melt over medium heat. Add the sweet potato and onion and sauté for 10 to 12 minutes, until softened. Next, add the apple, garlic, and red pepper flakes and sauté for 2 to 3 minutes more. Toss the kale and olive oil into the mix and sauté for about 3 minutes, until the kale is gently wilted. Season with salt to taste. Sprinkle with rosemary before removing from the pan.

TIME-SAVING TIP: Prepare the sweet potato the night before and cook the veggies and the apple in the morning. Toss in the sweet potato at the end to heat with all of the ingredients.

Vegetable Frittata

This vegetable and egg recipe is an easy-to-make weekend dish. It has five different vegetables—including onions, which are high in microbe-boosting inulin—and it looks vibrant and colorful on the table. Once you master the basic recipe, try experimenting with different vegetables, such as leeks and asparagus. Freeze in individual servings to pull out midweek when you need a hearty breakfast (or dinner!).

*SERVES 6

Ingredients

1 tablespoon olive oil or coconut oil

½ small yellow onion, diced

1 cup broccoli florets, cut into small pieces

½ zucchini, chopped

½ cup red bell pepper, chopped

2 cups spinach, loosely packed

8 large eggs

Sea salt and freshly ground black pepper to taste

Method

✳ PREHEAT THE OVEN to 350°F. In a 10-inch sauté pan or cast-iron skillet, add the olive oil and onion. Cook over medium heat for 2 to 3 minutes, until it begins to brown. Next, add the broccoli, zucchini, and bell pepper. Sauté for a few minutes, until soft and moist. Add in the spinach and cook for 1 to 2 minutes more, until slightly wilted. Remove the pan from the heat and allow the mixture to rest.

✳ IN A MEDIUM BOWL, beat the eggs and season with salt and black pepper. Add the eggs to the vegetable mixture, then place the sauté pan directly into the preheated oven (or transfer to a 9-inch pie plate before placing in the oven). Bake for 20 minutes, or until the eggs are well set and slightly browned. Slice into wedges and serve immediately.

Baked Avocado with Egg

For a low-sugar, high-protein breakfast, try this innovative morning meal. The combination of the healthy fats and lean protein will keep you feeling full and satisfied till lunchtime. It is also delicious topped with salsa and black beans.

*SERVES 2

Ingredients

    1 avocado
    2 large eggs
    Sea salt to taste
    Red pepper flakes to taste
    Chives, thinly sliced

NOTE: For one serving, divide the ingredients in half and keep the pit in the unused avocado half to prevent it from turning brown before consuming.

Method

✳ PREHEAT THE OVEN to 425°F. Slice the avocado in half and scoop out enough flesh from the avocado to make room for the eggs. Place the avocado halves in a small baking dish. Slowly crack the eggs into the avocado halves, ensuring that there is no overflow. Bake for 15 to 20 minutes, or until the whites are cooked through. Remove from the oven and season with salt, red pepper flakes, and chives.

Fruity Oats

Rolled oats are high in resistant starches and good for you and your microbes. Adding fruit to the cooking process takes them to the next level— not only does it taste delicious, it also eliminates the need for any additional sweeteners. Add in a spoon of nut butter or top with nuts and seeds for an even more filling breakfast.

*SERVES 2

Ingredients

    1 cup old-fashioned rolled oats
    2 cups water (or 1 cup water plus 1 cup plant-based milk)
    Fresh fruit, sliced (1 apple, 1 banana, 1 pear, or 1 peach), or 1 cup berries
    ¼ teaspoon sea salt

FLAVOR OPTIONS: ginger, cinnamon, nutmeg, lemon zest, or any other flavorings and spices

NUTRITION BOOSTS: nut butter, chopped nuts, seeds

Method

✳ COOK THE OATMEAL and water on the stove top according to the package directions. In the last 3 minutes, add in the fruit. Once cooked, the fruit should be soft and mix into the oats to form a semi-smooth consistency. Sprinkle with spices of your choice and top with a healthy protein and/or fat. Try flax, hemp, or chia seeds, a spoon of nut butter, or any combination of nuts.

Simple Chia Seed Pudding

This small seed produces big benefits. Chia seeds are a nutritional power-house filled with an easily digestible form of protein that's a rich source of

iron, magnesium, calcium, and phosphorus. Try this delicious chia seed pudding for breakfast, snack, or dessert. Mix it up by adding in some pureed berries or cocoa powder for variety.

*SERVES 4

Ingredients

    6 tablespoons chia seeds

    2 cups plant-based milk (almond, hemp, coconut)

    3 tablespoons pure maple syrup

    ½ teaspoon pure vanilla extract or vanilla powder

    Pinch of sea salt

ADD-INS: cinnamon, cardamom, pumpkin puree, lemon zest, maca

Method

✳ PLACE THE CHIA SEEDS, milk, maple syrup, vanilla, and salt in a medium bowl. Stir until well combined. Allow the mixture to sit for 30 minutes, whisking every 10 minutes until the mixture thickens. Place the bowl in the refrigerator and store for at least 2 hours or overnight. Check for the desired thickness and flavor. Adjust if needed. When ready to serve, spoon the pudding into bowls and top with fresh fruit. Keeps in the refrigerator up to 4 days.

VARIATIONS

BERRY CHIA SEED INFUSION: Add in 1 cup fresh or frozen pureed raspberries, plus 1 tablespoon lemon zest.

CHOCOLATE CHIA PUDDING: Mix in 2 tablespoons unsweetened cocoa powder or raw cacao powder.

Overnight Oats & Chia Seed Porridge

Overnight oats are a great option when you need a handy breakfast to go but you still want to eat according to the Live Dirty, Eat Clean Lifestyle. Add omega-rich chia seeds into the mix, and you have an easy-to-make, portable breakfast. Combine the ingredients in a jar at night, then in the

morning top with your favorite fruits and nutritional boosts. Eat right out of the jar or heat the mixture for a quick and warm meal.

*SERVES 1

Ingredients

½ cup gluten-free rolled oats

1 tablespoon chia seeds

½ cup DIY Nut Milk (page 213)

½ teaspoon ground cinnamon

½ teaspoon pure vanilla extract (omit if nut milk is flavored)

1 teaspoon maple syrup

TOPPINGS: fresh fruit (sliced bananas, apples, pears, chopped peaches, or fresh berries), nuts, shredded coconut, seeds

Method

✳ PLACE THE OATS, chia seeds, nut milk, cinnamon, vanilla, and maple syrup in a mason jar. Mix well. Place in the refrigerator overnight. In the morning, stir the mixture and add any desired toppings.

VARIATION: For a thicker and more filling meal, mash together 1 tablespoon almond butter and ½ banana. Place in the mason jar with the oat mixture to soak overnight.

Quinoa Berry Breakfast Bowl

Start your day right with a warm quinoa breakfast bowl. With all the essential amino acids and a big dose of plant-based protein, it's hard to beat the sustained energy you get from a meal filled with quinoa (technically a seed). Mix and match different fruits and nuts to prevent any breakfast bowl boredom.

*SERVES 1

Ingredients

¾ cup precooked quinoa (when prepping, use half water and
half DIY Nut Milk, page 213)

½ cup nut milk (use DIY Nut Milk, page 213, and add more
    for a creamier consistency)

½ teaspoon ground cinnamon

½ teaspoon pure vanilla extract

½ cup fresh blueberries

2 tablespoons shredded coconut

1 tablespoon sliced almonds, pecans, or sunflower seeds

Raw honey or maple syrup to taste (optional)

Method

✳ HEAT THE PRECOOKED QUINOA, nut milk, cinnamon, and vanilla in a small pot. Once warm, place in a bowl and top with the berries, shredded coconut, and nuts. Add more plant-based milk for extra creaminess.

Omega-Rich Granola

Homemade granola makes a quick breakfast, snack, or pick-me-up. This version is filled with healthy fats and less sugar than the packaged kinds. The recipe is forgiving, so feel free to mix and match with different combinations and flavors to create a unique batch each time. Add a few tablespoons as a crunchy topping to your smoothies, or enjoy with DIY Nut Milk (page 213) any time of day.

Ingredients

3 cups gluten-free old-fashioned oats

½ cup unsulfured shredded coconut

2 teaspoons ground cinnamon

1 teaspoon sea salt

1 cup nuts (walnuts, sliced almonds, pecans, hazelnuts, cashews)

1 cup seeds (sunflower seeds, pumpkin seeds)

½ cup maple syrup

1 teaspoon pure vanilla extract

2 tablespoons coconut oil, melted

1 cup unsweetened and unsulfured dried fruit (goji berries,
    cranberries, blueberries, or apricots) (optional)

Method

✻ PREHEAT THE OVEN to 325°F. Line two baking sheets with parchment paper. Put the oats, coconut, cinnamon, salt, nuts, and seeds in a big bowl. Pour the maple syrup, vanilla, and coconut oil over all of the ingredients. Mix with a spoon to coat evenly. Spread the mixture onto the baking sheets. Bake in the oven for 35 minutes, stirring after 20 minutes. Since oven temperatures may vary, check often as the granola can burn easily. Once evenly browned (about 35 minutes total baking time), remove the trays from the oven. Allow the granola to cool completely. Add the dried fruit, if using, and the omega-rich boost, if you desire, and mix.

VARIATION: For an omega-rich boost, sprinkle with hemp seeds, chia seeds, and flaxseeds while the granola is cooling and the tray is still hot.

Almond Flour Pancakes

These grain-free and gluten-free pancakes are also high in protein. Made with just a few ingredients, you can prepare them quickly in the morning and enjoy sustained energy for hours. Top with fresh berries or any seasonal fruit, and you'll be ready to take on the day.

*SERVES 4 TO 6

Ingredients

    3 large eggs

    2 tablespoons raw honey

    1 tablespoon water

    1½ cups almond flour

    ¼ to ½ teaspoon salt

    ¼ teaspoon baking soda

    Coconut oil for cooking

    1 teaspoon ground cinnamon

Method

✻ WHISK THE EGGS TOGETHER in a large bowl. Add in the honey and water. Mix until smooth. Next, add the almond flour, salt, and baking soda. Stir until the ingredients are thoroughly combined and a batter forms. Melt 1 tablespoon of coconut oil in a large skillet over low to medium heat. Once heated, place approximately 2 tablespoons of the batter at a time into the skillet, leaving enough space in between pancakes to flip. Cook until small bubbles form. Flip each pancake. Repeat with the remaining batter and add fresh oil as necessary. Sprinkle with the cinnamon and serve with fresh fruit. Yum!

Grain-Free Banana Pancakes

With only two ingredients plus a few seasonings, you can whip up these fruit-only sweetened pancakes in minutes. They are grain-free and sugar-free, but you won't be missing a thing in taste or flavor. For a more complete meal, top with berries and some chopped walnuts, almonds, or pecans.

*MAKES APPROXIMATELY TEN 3-INCH PANCAKES

Ingredients

1 banana

2 large eggs

¼ teaspoon ground cinnamon

¼ teaspoon sea salt

¼ teaspoon baking powder

Coconut oil for greasing pan

Method

✳ MASH THE BANANA in a medium bowl. Whisk the eggs in a separate small bowl, then mix with the mashed banana. Once the mixture is smooth, add in the cinnamon, salt, and baking powder. Heat the pan over medium-high heat and lightly grease the pan with coconut oil. Once the pan is hot, drop 2 tablespoons at a time into the pan, cooking for 30 seconds to 1 minute on each side, until browned around the edges. Eat immediately. Enjoy!

Banana Blueberry Flaxseed Muffins

These grain-free, fiber-rich morsels are a great pre-exercise snack or on-the-go breakfast. Forget about the store-bought versions and prepare a batch of these microbe-friendly muffins early in the week. They freeze beautifully and can be pulled out in a pinch whenever you need a quick and nourishing addition to your morning.

*MAKES 12 MUFFINS

Ingredients

Coconut oil to grease muffin pans

1 cup mashed bananas (3 large ripe bananas)

3 large eggs

2 tablespoons raw honey

2 tablespoons coconut oil, melted

¾ cup almond flour

¼ cup coconut flour

¾ teaspoon baking soda

½ teaspoon salt

1 tablespoon ground flaxseeds

½ cup fresh or frozen blueberries

Method

✳ GREASE A 12-CUP MUFFIN TIN with coconut oil and set aside. In a large bowl, mash the bananas. Add the eggs and mix. Next, add the honey and coconut oil and mix well. In a separate medium bowl, mix the almond flour, coconut flour, baking soda, salt, and flaxseeds. Pour the dry ingredients into the wet ingredients and stir. Once mixed, add the frozen blueberries; add the blueberries last to prevent the batter from turning blue! Gently mix. Pour the batter into the prepared muffin tin and place in the oven for 30 minutes. Check after 25 minutes as oven temperatures can vary. Enjoy with Coconut Milk Kefir (page 263) for a microbe-boosting breakfast.

SMOOTHIES, JUICES & OTHER LIQUIDS

Live Dirty, Eat Clean Signature Smoothie

This smoothie is the perfect solution when you need a little hydration after a sweaty workout or when you want to clean out the digestive pipes with healthy fiber in a liquid form. It's the perfect breakfast-to-go option. The coconut water contains tons of electrolytes, while the berries and greens are loaded with microbe-friendly indigestible plant fiber. Enzymes such as bromelain in the pineapple help with digestion, and the banana is a good source of inulin. Need a more filling smoothie? Swap out the coconut water for fermented coconut kefir.

*SERVES 2

Ingredients

1 cup coconut water (or Coconut Milk Kefir, page 263)

2 handfuls spinach

1 cup fresh or frozen blueberries

4 to 5 chunks (about ½ cup) fresh or frozen pineapple

1 banana

Method

✳ PLACE THE COCONUT WATER, spinach, blueberries, pineapple, and banana in the bowl of a high-speed blender, blend for 1 minute, and enjoy.

Apple Pie Green Smoothie

What do you get when you mix the tastes and flavors of apple pie with greens? Answer: an amazing glass of goodness that will keep you energized and happy for hours. The addition of tahini gives this a touch of creaminess, while the uncooked rolled oats add a bit of heartiness and extra fiber for days when you need a little more than blended-up berries.

*SERVES 1

Ingredients

¾ to 1 cup almond milk (use less for a thicker smoothie)

2 handfuls spinach

1 apple, cored and cubed

1 small banana, sliced and frozen

1 tablespoon tahini (cashew or almond butter works, too)

1 teaspoon ground cinnamon

Dash of ground nutmeg (optional)

2 tablespoons old-fashioned oats

Mix-and-Match Toppings: chopped apples, chia seeds, hemp seeds, walnuts, pecans

Method

✳ MIX THE ALMOND MILK, spinach, apple, banana, tahini, cinnamon, nutmeg, and oats in the container of a high-speed blender and blend until smooth. Then garnish with your favorite toppings.

Creamy Sweet Potato Smoothie

Sweet potatoes are the perfect nutrient-dense food to help stave off sugar cravings. This creamy smoothie is loaded with antioxidants and is also a great source of plant-based energy. Enjoy first thing in the morning or serve it in smaller portions for a satisfying dessert. The warming anti-inflammatory spices are perfect on a crisp fall or cold winter day.

*SERVES 1 FOR BREAKFAST OR 2 FOR DESSERT

Ingredients

¾ to 1 cup unsweetened almond milk (see DIY Nut Milk, page 213)

½ cup cooked sweet potato

1 small banana, sliced and frozen

1 tablespoon almond butter (cashew butter or sunflower butter works, too)

½ teaspoon grated fresh ginger root

Sprinkle of ground cinnamon, or to taste

Toppings: hemp seeds and additional cinnamon (optional)

Method

✳ PLACE THE ALMOND MILK, sweet potato, banana, almond butter, ginger, and cinnamon in the container of a high-speed blender and blend until smooth. Add the toppings, if you wish. Sip and savor.

VARIATION: For an added microbiome boost, add ½ teaspoon grated fresh turmeric.

For a thicker smoothie, add ice.

Blueberry Bliss Smoothie

Filled with lots of nutrient-dense ingredients, this beautiful blue meal in a glass is sure to help you start your day out on the right note. With blueberries, almonds, spinach, and avocados all in one place, your body—and microbes—will be thanking you all morning long.

*SERVES 1

Ingredients

    1 cup almond milk (see DIY Nut Milk, page 213)
    2 handfuls spinach
    ½ small avocado
    ½ banana, sliced and frozen
    1 cup frozen blueberries (or any berry combination works),
        plus more for garnish
    2 teaspoons hemp seeds

Method

✳ PLACE THE ALMOND MILK and spinach in the container of a high-speed blender and puree until smooth. Add the avocado, banana, and blueberries and blend until the desired consistency is reached. Top with additional blueberries and hemp seeds.

VARIATION: Sweeten with raw honey or fresh pitted dates in place of the banana.

Everything but the Kitchen Sink Smoothie

The beauty of smoothies is that you don't really need a recipe. Just open up your refrigerator and create your own combination of flavors depending on what you have on hand. As long as you make sure that it's nutritionally balanced, you can whip up your creation in no time.

Follow this general formula:

✳ PICK A LIQUID BASE: plant-based milk, coconut water, coconut kefir, green tea, or even plain filtered water.

✳ ADD A FEW HANDFULS OF LEAFY GREENS: spinach, romaine lettuce, kale, Swiss chard, dandelion greens. (Challenge yourself to make it super green. For picky eaters, start with just a few greens and gradually increase as the palate adjusts.)

✳ INCLUDE SOME FRUIT (fresh or frozen): berries, banana, apple, pineapple, mango, melon, or pear.

✳ DON'T FORGET FATS AND PROTEIN: nuts, nut butter, seeds, coconut oil, coconut meat, avocado, flaxseed oil.

✳ BLEND!

Creamy Turmeric Latte

Turmeric is the vibrant orange-yellow spice affectionately known as the magic sword against inflammation, birthed in India and crowned centuries ago as one of the great dosha balancers in Ayurvedic medicine. With all the healing benefits, you can taste the inherent goodness with each sip. It is just as delicious as it is nutritious.

*SERVES 1

Ingredients

1 cup unsweetened almond or coconut milk

1 heaping tablespoon grated fresh turmeric root (or use approximately
   2 teaspoons turmeric paste—see below)

1 tablespoon grated fresh ginger root
   (or 1 teaspoon ground)

1 teaspoon ground cinnamon

1 tablespoon coconut oil or ghee

Raw honey to taste

NOTE: To make the turmeric paste, combine 2 parts turmeric powder with 1 part boiling water. Mix and store any extra in the refrigerator for up to 5 days.

Method

✳ GENTLY WARM THE ALMOND or coconut milk in a small saucepan over medium heat. Do not boil. Add the turmeric, ginger, and cinnamon. Add the coconut oil, combine, and heat together until the coconut oil has melted. Use a wire whisk or immersion blender to create foam. Continue to stir until frothy and heated through. Stir in honey to taste. Sip, savor, and enjoy.

DIY Nut Milk

Homemade nut milk is budget-friendly and easy to make, plus most commercial varieties contain ingredients that are questionable for microbial health. Once you make your first batch, you'll wonder why it took you so long to upgrade your plant-based milk to homemade. All you need is a quart-size jar, a nut milk bag (or an old T-shirt), and a blender. No sugar. No additives. Just pure ingredients.

Ingredients

> 1 cup nuts (almonds, cashews, Brazil nuts, hazelnuts—
>   all work great)
> 3 to 4 cups filtered water (use less water for a creamier milk)
> 1 to 2 dates, as a sweetener (optional)
> Pinch of sea salt

Method

✳ SOAK THE NUTS FOR at least 6 hours or overnight with enough water to cover. (Cashews only need 4 to 6 hours.) Drain the water and place the soaked nuts in the bowl of a blender with the filtered water. Blend for a few minutes. For a touch of sweetness, add in dates, if desired. Toss in the salt. Blend again until smooth. Pour the mixture into a nut milk bag and squeeze out all of the liquid over a bowl. Discard the pulp and place the milk in a mason jar or airtight glass container. Store in the refrigerator for up to 3 days.

VARIATIONS: Once you get comfortable with the basic recipe, feel free to add pure vanilla extract, ground cinnamon, turmeric, cocoa powder, or any other flavors and spices you desire.

Green Colada

A Live Dirty, Eat Clean "mocktail." While your friends are lounging with a cocktail in hand, whip up a refreshing Green Colada instead. You'll get a hefty dose of fiber, vitamins, minerals, antioxidants, and digestive enzymes, too, with no nasty hangover.

*SERVES 1

Ingredients

1 cucumber

3 to 4 kale leaves

4 to 5 chunks (about ½ cup) fresh or frozen pineapple

1 handful cilantro

½ cup coconut water

Raw honey to taste

1 teaspoon pure vanilla extract

OPTIONAL: Freeze the pineapple ahead of time for a thicker consistency and frothy texture.

Method

✴ PLACE THE CUCUMBER, kale leaves, pineapple, cilantro, coconut water, honey, and vanilla in the bowl of a high-speed blender and blend for 1 minute.

Green Lemonade

Leafy greens are the most important—and the most underrepresented— ingredient in the American diet. Try drinking them as a quick and easy alternative—or addition—to eating them. Although the fiber content with juicing is less than with blending, this lemonade still provides lots of nutrients and a great alternative to water that's still super healthy.

Ingredients

1 head romaine lettuce

1 large lemon, peeled

4 or 5 kale leaves

1 handful spinach

2 stalks of celery

1 cucumber, peeled

1 pear

1-inch slice fresh ginger root

OPTIONAL ADD-INS: 1 lime, peeled; 1 apple in place of pear; handful of parsley; fresh mint

Method

✳ PLACE THE LETTUCE, lemon, kale, spinach, celery, cucumber, pear, and ginger in a juicer. Add the optional ingredients as desired. Then sip and savor your green goodness.

Lemonchia Coconut Water

For a fun way to keep your hydration levels up, add chia seeds and a squeeze of lemon to your coconut water. Filled with plant-based protein and healthy omega-3 fatty acids, a Lemonchia Coconut Water will take the edge off your hunger and keep you satiated longer than regular water. The lemon is a great detoxifier to include in your new gut-friendly routine.

*SERVES 2

Ingredients

1½ tablespoons chia seeds

2 cups coconut water

½ lemon

1 teaspoon raw honey (optional)

Method

✳ ADD THE CHIA SEEDS to the coconut water and stir or shake. Let the mixture stand for at least 15 minutes to allow the seeds to absorb the water. Squeeze the lemon into the water mixture and shake the mixture again. If desired, add the honey.

Colorful Kale Salad

This salad is going to be one of your new favorites. Lacinato kale, also known as dinosaur kale, isn't as tough as curly kale and works great in raw salads. The colorful dish not only tastes good but is also filled with tons of indigestible plant fiber to feed your microbes.

*SERVES 4

Ingredients

> 1 bunch lacinato (a.k.a. dinosaur) kale, thick stems removed and
>   leaves thinly sliced
>
> 4 cups shredded red cabbage (about 1 small head, cored and sliced)
>
> 2 navel oranges or clementines, peeled and segmented
>
> 1 small red onion, thinly sliced
>
> 1 large red bell pepper, cored, seeded, and thinly sliced
>
> ⅓ cup sunflower seeds
>
> 1 tablespoon Dijon mustard
>
> ¼ cup freshly squeezed lemon juice
>
> ¼ cup olive oil
>
> 2 tablespoons chopped fresh basil (optional)
>
> 1 tablespoon maple syrup
>
> Salt and freshly ground black pepper to taste

Method

✳ IN A LARGE BOWL, combine the kale, cabbage, orange segments, onion, bell pepper, and sunflower seeds. In a small bowl, whisk together the mustard, lemon juice, olive oil, basil if desired, and maple syrup. Season with salt and black pepper. Pour the dressing over the kale mixture and toss to coat. Serve immediately. Store extra dressing in the refrigerator and store any extra salad for up to 2 days.

Cabbage Crunch

Cabbage is one of the Live Dirty, Eat Clean prebiotic superstars and a delicious way to feed both you and your microbes. This salad actually tastes just as good the next day. Make it on the weekend, and you will have an already prepared and delicious lunch to enjoy for a few days.

*SERVES 6 TO 8

Ingredients

DRESSING

3 tablespoons olive oil

2 teaspoons toasted sesame oil

¼ cup freshly squeezed lime juice

Zest of 1 lime

1 tablespoon mirin

1 tablespoon raw honey

Sea salt to taste

SALAD

½ medium red cabbage, finely shredded

1 large green cabbage, finely shredded

2 large carrots, peeled and shredded

3 green onions, thinly sliced

⅓ cup chopped fresh cilantro

2 tablespoons toasted sesame seeds

½ cup crushed peanuts (cashews work, too)

Method

✳ WHISK ALL OF THE dressing ingredients in a separate small bowl. Let stand. Combine the red cabbage, green cabbage, carrots, green onions, and cilantro in a large bowl. Pour the dressing over mixture, then add in toasted sesame seeds. Toss again. Allow to marinate for 30 minutes. Add the crushed peanuts to salad before serving. Store unused salad and dressing separately in the refrigerator for up to 2 days. Mix before serving.

Sliced Kale & Brussels Sprouts Salad

This salad is not just another kale salad. It's an innovative way to get your daily dose of greens and receive the power-packed nutrients of two of the Live Dirty, Eat Clean favorite greens. The raw Brussels sprouts add a distinct flavor that pairs perfectly with the crunchy almonds and the lemon-shallot vinaigrette.

*SERVES 6

Ingredients

SALAD

4 cups lacinato kale, loosely packed

4 cups Brussels sprouts, loosely packed

½ cup sliced almonds, toasted

DRESSING

¼ cup freshly squeezed lemon juice

1 tablespoon Dijon mustard

1 tablespoon chopped shallots

1 tablespoon lemon zest

1 tablespoon maple syrup

¼ cup olive oil

Sea salt and freshly ground black pepper to taste

Method

✳ REMOVE AND DISCARD the stalks from the kale. Roll the leaves, and then slice into thin strips. Halve the Brussels sprouts, discard the ends, then finely grate or shred them with a knife into thin slices. Assemble the kale and Brussels sprouts in a large bowl.

✳ FOR THE DRESSING, mix together the lemon juice, mustard, shallots, lemon zest, and maple syrup. Whisk until well combined. Slowly add in olive oil and mix. Season with salt and pepper. Drizzle the dressing over the kale and Brussels sprouts. Toss to coat. Add sliced almonds and mix. Enjoy!

VARIATION: Add pomegranate seeds and chopped chickpeas for a twist on this simple salad.

Quinoa Tabbouleh Salad

This is a modern take on an old favorite. Traditionally, tabbouleh is made with bulgur wheat, but this version is Live Dirty, Eat Clean–approved with quinoa, which is gluten-free and also contains a healthy dose of plant-based protein. Tabbouleh is satisfying as a main dish served on a bed of greens, or it can be used as a filling in a brown rice or collard wrap (see Rainbow Collard Green Wraps, page 229). Make this dish in advance for an easy grab-and-go option.

*SERVES 6 TO 8

Ingredients

1 cup uncooked quinoa, rinsed and drained

2 cups water

1 cup peeled and chopped cucumbers

½ cup chopped scallions

1 cup chopped fresh parsley

¼ cup chopped fresh mint

1 cup quartered grape (or cherry) tomatoes

Sea salt and freshly ground black pepper to taste

¼ cup olive oil

¼ cup freshly squeezed lemon juice

1 teaspoon minced garlic

Method

✳ IN A SMALL POT, combine the quinoa and water (or use half vegetable broth for a boost of flavor). Bring to a boil, cover, and reduce the heat to low. Simmer until done, about 15 minutes. Chill thoroughly, at least 30 minutes. Add the cucumbers, scallions, parsley, mint, and tomatoes to the quinoa. Next, season with salt and pepper to taste. In a separate small bowl, whisk the olive oil, lemon juice, and garlic until blended. Add to the quinoa and veggies and mix until thoroughly combined. Chill before serving.

Roasted Root Vegetable Salad

A warming salad that feels good to eat no matter what the temperature is outside. The flavor of the balsamic maple vinaigrette adds just the right amount of sweetness to the mix. Roast the vegetables in advance and serve them at room temperature the next day, or enjoy right out of the oven for a meal that will make you feel rooted and grounded with every bite.

*SERVES 4 TO 6

Ingredients

VEGETABLES

4 cups root vegetable mixture, cubed or sliced in sticks
  (carrots, parsnip, beets, squash, anything goes)

Olive oil for coating the root vegetables

Sea salt and freshly ground black pepper to taste

¼ cup chopped fresh parsley

8 cups mixed greens (can use spinach, spring mix, mache, arugula)

Topping: dried cranberries and walnuts

DRESSING

¼ cup olive oil

¼ cup balsamic vinegar

1 tablespoon water

1 tablespoon maple syrup

2 teaspoons Dijon mustard

1 tablespoon chopped fresh herbs (optional; thyme, parsley,
  and rosemary work well)

Sea salt and freshly ground black pepper to taste

Method

✻ PREHEAT THE OVEN to 400°F. Line a rimmed baking sheet with parchment paper. Cut the root vegetables into either cubes or sticks and coat with the olive oil, salt, pepper, and parsley. Place in a single layer on the baking sheet and roast for 35 to 40 minutes, or until golden brown around the edges and crispy. (The roasting time depends on the thickness of the sliced veggies.) Turn over once halfway through cooking. Remove the veggies from the oven and cool slightly. While cooling, make the dressing by whisking together the olive oil, vinegar, water, maple syrup, mustard, herbs if using, salt, and pepper in a small bowl. Place the vegetables on a bed of greens. Add some dried cranberries and walnuts and drizzle with the balsamic maple dressing. Store extra dressing in the refrigerator for up to 5 days. Serve warm or at room temperature.

Mason Jar Salads

Imagine opening up your refrigerator and seeing ready-to-go salads all lined up just waiting to be eaten. While an official recipe to create a mason jar salad isn't really necessary, there is a bit of an art to building the perfect mason jar salad to avoid ending up eating a soggy mess. (Hint: it's all about the layering.)

Mason Jar Size: Use a widemouthed jar that's easy to fill . . . and easy to dig into. The pint size is perfect for an individual salad and is deceptively bigger and more filling than it looks. If packed with nutrient-dense ingredients, it should keep you full for hours. For larger salads, use the quart size.

Dressing: Wet ingredients go on the bottom. By keeping the mason jar upright, the dressing won't mix with the rest of the salad until you're ready to eat it. Try using hummus or pesto instead of traditional salad dressing. Anything else with a marinade should stay close to the bottom as well.

Hard Vegetables: Veggies such as carrots, cucumbers, peppers, celery, onion, zucchini, fennel, and cooked beets can be layered on top of the dressing because they are not as absorbent.

Softer Fruits & Veggies: In the middle, place the more absorbent veggies, such as avocado, tomatoes, berries, or citrus fruits. (If using avocado, add a squeeze of lemon to prevent browning.)

Grains, Beans, Nuts, Seeds & Proteins: These nutritional powerhouses stay fresh closer to the top. The nuts and seeds maintain their crunch if placed right below the top layer. (Note: Beans can also go near the bottom.)

Greens: Last but not least, fill the remaining part of the jar with as much leafy greens as you can possibly fit in (or bring along some extras to make sure to get your daily fill of gorgeous greens).

Storing: Make sure to screw the lid on as tightly as possible so that your salad can last up to 4 days.

Eating: When it comes time to eat your gorgeous salad, either shake it up and go for it straight from the jar, or pull out a bowl and do "the flip": turn the mason jar upside down into a dish and end up with the greens on the bottom and all the other ingredients on top, including the dressing.

INGREDIENT INSPIRATION

Use your imagination and try not to get stuck in the idea of having to follow a recipe exactly.

Here are a few ideas meant to inspire:

Raid the refrigerator for leftovers (or intentionally make extra). Roast lots of veggies at the beginning of the week, make some extra protein, and cook a batch of quinoa or brown rice. Then, when it comes time to filling all the jars, mix and match to create a variety of perfectly balanced lunches to keep things interesting all week long. (No two salads are alike, so you can say good-bye to lunchtime boredom.)

Pick a theme. Think Mediterranean, Mexican, Asian-inspired, or Italian, and then build your salad with all the flavors and ingredients accordingly.

Deconstruct a salad you already make. As an example, take the Colorful Kale Salad (page 216) and then layer all of the ingredients instead of mixing them together.

Get ideas from other dishes. The Zucchini Pasta with Pesto & Cherry Tomatoes (page 229) is a tasty option. Just layer the pesto on the bottom, and then add the zucchini noodles plus lots of tomatoes. To make it more of a salad, add in other crunchy veggies, such as carrots and red bell peppers.

DIPS & DRESSINGS

Guac-Kale-Mole

Guac-Kale-Mole brings guacamole to a whole new level in taste and nutrition. How can you go wrong when you mix kale with avocado? The key is to soften the kale and massage it first with a drop of olive oil so that it blends well with the creamy avocado. Make the guacamole by hand, and then process the kale and blend it into the avocado mixture. This is likely to become your new microbiome-friendly snack.

*SERVES 6

Ingredients

2 to 3 avocados, pitted and peeled

Freshly squeezed juice of 1 lime

¼ cup chopped red onion

½ clove garlic, chopped

½ to 1 jalapeño pepper, seeded and chopped

2 tablespoons chopped fresh cilantro

¼ teaspoon ground cumin

Sea salt to taste

4 to 5 large kale leaves, stalks removed and discarded

Drop of olive oil for massaging the kale

Method

✳ MIX AND MASH the avocados, lime juice, onion, garlic, jalapeño, cilantro, cumin, and salt together in a bowl to the desired consistency. Massage the kale with a drop of olive oil to soften it, then process in the bowl of a high-speed blender or food processor. Once smooth, add the kale to the guacamole. Serve with sliced-up crunchy vegetables such as jicama, carrots, and red bell pepper.

Artichoke & Spinach Dip

With artichoke as the main player in this dish, you'll fill up on a hefty dose of inulin. Eat this with jicama and carrots or spread on Chickpea Herbed Crackers (page 257) for the perfect Live Dirty, Eat Clean combination of microbiome-friendly players.

*SERVES 2 TO 4

Ingredients

¾ cup artichoke hearts (ideally fresh, or use artichokes from a glass
   container in water)

1 cup baby spinach

½ cup pine nuts

1 teaspoon freshly squeezed lemon juice

1 clove garlic

1 teaspoon light miso

¼ cup olive oil

Sea salt and freshly ground black pepper to taste

Method

❋ PLACE THE ARTICHOKE HEARTS, spinach, pine nuts, lemon juice, garlic, and miso in the bowl of a food processor. Drizzle in olive oil while food processor is mixing. Pulse until smooth. Add salt and pepper to taste.

Cashew "Cheese" Spread

A great alternative to dairy cheese spreads, this cashew spread is a creamy, dreamy accompaniment to a collard wrap (see Rainbow Collard Green Wraps, page 229) and also great on Chickpea Herbed Crackers (page 257).

Ingredients

1½ cups soaked cashews (soak for around 3 hours)

2 tablespoons freshly squeezed lemon juice

1 teaspoon sea salt

1 teaspoon light miso (or 2 teaspoons nutritional yeast)

1 teaspoon onion powder

1 to 3 tablespoons water

Method

❋ RINSE THE SOAKED CASHEWS WELL. Place the cashews, lemon juice, salt, miso, and onion powder in the bowl of a food processor. Pulse. Add water as needed. The texture should be soft like cream cheese. It's that simple!

Creamy Ginger Tahini Dressing

This flavorful dressing is a little sweet and a little salty. Use it for salads, collard wraps (see Rainbow Collard Green Wraps, page 229), on bowls (see

How to Build a Bowl, page 226), or over warm grains. A little bit goes a long way.

Ingredients

¼ cup tahini

2 tablespoons rice vinegar

2 teaspoons sesame oil

¼ cup water

¼ cup gluten-free tamari

1 tablespoon maple syrup

1 tablespoon freshly grated ginger

½ teaspoon red pepper flakes

Method

✳ WHISK THE TAHINI, rice vinegar, sesame oil, water, tamari, maple syrup, ginger, and red pepper flakes together until smooth and well combined. Adjust with liquids or seasonings if necessary.

Basic Lemon Vinaigrette

Here is a dressing that will work on all of your green salads that can be made in a variety of ways using Live Dirty, Eat Clean–approved ingredients. Learn the basic method and then experiment by mixing in some chopped shallots or garlic for their flavor and health benefits.

Ingredients

¼ cup freshly squeezed lemon juice

1 tablespoon Dijon mustard

2 teaspoons maple syrup

1 tablespoon chopped fresh herbs (basil, oregano, parsley)

2 teaspoons lemon zest

¼ cup olive oil

Sea salt and freshly ground black pepper to taste

Method

✳ IN A SMALL BOWL, whisk together the lemon juice, mustard, and maple syrup. Add in the fresh herbs and lemon zest (plus shallots or garlic, if experimenting). Slowly add the olive oil to the dressing mixture and blend until well combined. Season with salt and pepper to taste. Pour over the salad and toss to coat. Store the remaining dressing in the refrigerator until the next salad (up to 5 days).

MAINS

Build a Bowl

If you feel stressed about preparing a delicious and nourishing meal after a long day, there's a simple solution: a genius blend of hearty ingredients assembled in a bowl—no recipe required. All you need is to set aside some time to shop and then prep your food in advance. (Proclaim Sunday "kitchen fun day"—good music, good conversation, and lots of chopping, steaming, stirring, grilling, and roasting.) When you arrive home exhausted and hungry, all your food will be waiting to be thrown together in a bowl. You'll never have to wonder what's for dinner again. Bowls are like the "little black dress" of meal planning, filled with staples such as whole grains, protein, healthy fats, and tons of veggies. Just add a few key "accessories" to spice it up.

Here's a simple guide to building balanced, nourishing, and delicious meals in a bowl.

How to Build a Bowl

To make sure that the bowls are balanced in flavor, texture, and nutrition, choose at least one ingredient from each category. (Bonus points for going heavy on the veggies!)

Start with a base of leafy greens: spinach, kale, shredded Brussels sprouts, Swiss chard, mustard greens, arugula, bok choy, pea shoots, or lettuce

Add unlimited raw, roasted, steamed, or grilled veggies: carrots, peppers, beets, roasted eggplant, asparagus, Brussels sprouts, broccoli, cauliflower, bean sprouts, green beans, mushrooms, zucchini, tomatoes, shredded cabbage, onion, jicama

Toss in a grain or starch: quinoa, brown rice, wild rice, butternut squash, sweet potatoes, soba (buckwheat) noodles

Include protein: chickpeas, black beans, lentils, salmon, tuna, grilled chicken, edamame, veggie burgers, hard-boiled eggs

Don't forget the healthy fats: seeds, nuts, avocado, drizzle of pumpkin, coconut, or olive oil

Top it off with dressings/sauces: hummus, lemon/lime squeeze and olive oil, tahini, salsa, pesto, miso ginger sauce, tamari

Not sure where to start? Pick a theme for every night of the week. Try Mediterranean with brown rice, lentils, and spinach as your main ingredients. Or Mexican, and fill your bowl with grilled chicken, black beans, and a mango salsa. Go for a more Asian-inspired meal with tofu, brown rice, edamame, red bell peppers, and broccoli. Choose roasted veggies and quinoa to pair with a warm tahini sauce. Anything goes. Just be willing to get a little creative.

When it's time to eat dinner each night, pull out some large bowls and let everyone mix and match their ingredients. Some like spicy foods, others prefer simple combos, and one might be all plant-based while another may need animal protein. The possibilities are endless. No two bowls are alike. Everybody is happy . . . without a recipe.

Live Dirty, Eat Clean Signature Bowl

With the Live Dirty, Eat Clean Plan, you'll learn to toss together meals that are perfectly balanced and filled with microbe-boosting ingredients in no time. Use this bowl as an example to inspire you to assemble your own nourishing creations.

*MAKES 2 LARGE BOWLS

Ingredients

1 to 2 cups cooked brown rice or quinoa

2 to 3 tablespoons coconut oil or olive oil

1 red onion, thinly sliced

4 carrots, peeled and thinly sliced

3 stalks celery, thinly sliced

1 cup Curry & Turmeric Roasted Cauliflower (page 240)

1 cup cooked chickpeas

1 bunch kale, stalks removed and discarded and leaves sliced thin

2 cups baby spinach

1 cup cherry tomatoes, sliced in half

¼ cup dried Turkish apricots, chopped (or raisins, dried cranberries, or dried cherries)

¼ cup toasted pecans, chopped

1 bunch of fresh parsley, chopped (about ½ cup)

DRESSING

½-inch piece of fresh ginger, peeled and minced

2 tablespoons freshly squeezed lemon juice

1 teaspoon raw honey

1 teaspoon Dijon mustard

¼ teaspoon red pepper flakes

¼ cup olive oil

Method

✳ REHEAT THE PRECOOKED BROWN RICE. Divide the rice into two separate bowls. Heat a large pan over medium-high heat and add the coconut oil. Stir in onion, carrots, and celery. Sauté the vegetables for 3 to 4 minutes, until they begin to soften and brown. In the last minute, toss in the cauliflower and chickpeas. Next, add the kale to the mix and allow the kale to slightly wilt for about 1 minute. Remove the pan from the heat and add the baby spinach and tomatoes. Place the sautéed mixture over the brown rice. Add in the dried apricots.

✳ TO MAKE THE DRESSING, mix together the ginger, lemon juice, honey, mustard, and red pepper flakes in a small mixing bowl. Slowly whisk in the olive oil to form an emulsion. Drizzle the dressing over the bowls. Toss lightly. Top with toasted pecans and fresh parsley. Save any remaining dressing in the refrigerator for up to 4 days.

Rainbow Collard Green Wraps

Collard leaves are great for your microbes and can take the place of a traditional grain-based wrap. Use this list for inspiration and then fill the wrap with any of the Live Dirty, Eat Clean–approved ingredients on the plan. Have fun and get creative.

Ingredients

Sliced or shredded colorful vegetables: cabbage, carrots, beets, jicama, red bell peppers, yellow bell peppers, broccoli sprouts, pea shoots, cucumber, avocado, zucchini, summer squash

Collard greens

Spread: hummus, pesto (see Zucchini Pasta with Pesto & Cherry Tomatoes, below), cashew cheese (see Cashew "Cheese" Spread, page 224), or mashed avocado (see page 222 for dips and dressing option)

Precooked quinoa or brown rice (optional)

Method

✳ SLICE OR SHRED the vegetables into thin strips using either a mandolin or a slicer, or by cutting them by hand. Lay all of the strips out on a plate or cutting board. Wash and dry the collard leaves. Shave down the thick stalk and then flip the collard leaves over. Place the moist ingredients in the middle of each leaf and spread (use avocado, cashew cheese, hummus), then fill the leaves with all the colors of the rainbow. Add in quinoa for a more filling wrap. Fold the sides in first and then roll up like a burrito. Eat whole or slice in half.

Zucchini Pasta with Pesto & Cherry Tomatoes

Zucchini "pasta" is an amazingly delicious substitute for regular pasta that will leave you feeling great—and not bloated—after eating it. There are multiple ways to prepare it so that you won't ever become tired of this easy-to-make favorite. The secret is in the sauce. Try this dairy-free and deli-

cious pesto for starters. *The pesto can be made the night before for an easy and refreshing meal.*

Ingredients

4 zucchinis

2 cups fresh basil leaves, tightly packed

½ cup walnuts or pine nuts

1 clove garlic, coarsely chopped

¼ to ½ cup olive oil, added until desired consistency is reached

½ teaspoon sea salt

Freshly ground black pepper to taste

1 cup cherry tomatoes, chopped

Method

✳ FOR THE "PASTA," use a julienne peeler or knife to make long thin slices of zucchini. If you own a spiralizer, that's a less labor intensive way to make the noodles.

✳ COMBINE THE BASIL, nuts, and garlic in the bowl of a food processor and blend until coarsely ground. Slowly drizzle in the olive oil and process. Add enough olive oil to keep it moist. Next, add the salt and the pepper to taste. Cover the zucchini with the pesto and top with the chopped tomatoes. Store the remaining pesto in a tightly sealed container in the refrigerator for up to 4 days.

White Bean Vegetarian Chili

Who doesn't love a bowl of piping hot chili? When it's made with fresh microbiome-friendly ingredients, it's a no-brainer. Prepare the beans in advance, then cook up a pot of this warming chili. Serve with a simple green salad as a side, or add in some brown rice or quinoa for a heartier meal.

Ingredients

2 tablespoons olive oil

1 onion, minced

1 teaspoon dried oregano

1 teaspoon ground cumin

1 tablespoon chili powder

½ teaspoon cinnamon

1 jalapeño pepper, cored and seeded

2 or 3 cloves garlic

2 small zucchinis, chopped

1 large red or orange bell pepper, cored, seeded, and diced

1 medium sweet potato, cut into ¼-inch cubes

2 cups diced fresh tomatoes with juice

1 cup water

1 cup vegetable stock (plus more as needed to achieve desired
    thickness)

One 7-ounce jar tomato paste (choose glass over canned,
    if possible)

1 teaspoon sea salt

4 cups cooked white beans

1 avocado, diced, for garnish

1 bunch cilantro, chopped, for garnish

Dash of hot sauce (optional), for garnish

Method

✳ IN A LARGE STOCKPOT, heat 1 tablespoon olive oil over medium-high heat.
Add the onion and sauté it. Once the onion begins to sweat, add the oregano,
cumin, chili powder, cinnamon, jalapeño, and garlic. Cook for 1 to 2 minutes, until
softened. Next, add the remaining 1 tablespoon of olive oil, the zucchini, bell
pepper, sweet potato, tomatoes, water, stock, tomato paste, salt, and cooked
beans. Bring the mixture to a boil. Reduce the heat to a simmer. Cover and cook
for 35 to 40 minutes, or until all of the vegetables are soft. Serve hot and top each
bowl with avocado and cilantro. For a little heat, add a dash of hot sauce.

NOTE: This recipe works with any combination of beans.

Grain-Free & Vegan Veggie Burgers

*This is a grain-free, gluten-free, and dairy-free veggie burger that is
not meant to taste like meat. Filled with lots of vegetables and even more*

flavor, enjoy these on Meatless Monday or any day of the week. They are a little more complicated than some of the other recipes, but the effort is well worth it.

*MAKES 10 PATTIES

Ingredients

1 tablespoon olive oil

½ medium head cauliflower, cored and chopped into
    small pieces (about 3 cups chopped)

½ medium yellow onion, chopped into small pieces
    (about ¾ cup chopped)

1 stalk celery, peeled and chopped

1 large carrot, peeled and chopped

1 medium sweet potato, peeled and shredded
    (about 1½ cups shredded)

2 cloves garlic, peeled and chopped

1 teaspoon ground cumin

½ teaspoon dried oregano

½ teaspoon sea salt

¼ teaspoon freshly ground black pepper

¼ cup sunflower seeds

¼ cup sesame seeds

2 tablespoons ground flaxseeds

1 flax egg (1 tablespoon ground flaxseed soaked in 2 tablespoons warm
    water—let sit for 10 minutes)

Method

✳ HEAT THE OLIVE OIL in a large skillet over medium heat. Add the cauliflower, onion, celery, and carrot. Cook for 5 to 7 minutes, until just tender. Add the sweet potato and garlic to the pan. Mix the veggies thoroughly and then add the cumin, oregano, salt, and pepper. Mix well and allow the veggies to cook for 5 minutes more, until tender. Remove the pan from the heat and allow the veggie mixture to cool.

✳ WHILE THE VEGGIES are cooling, grind the sunflower seeds and sesame seeds in the bowl of a food processor, making sure not to overprocess. Pour the seed mixture into a separate bowl and mix in the ground flaxseeds. Set aside.

Next, place the veggie mixture in the food processor and pulse the veggies until all of the larger chunks are gone. Add in the seed/flax mixture and pulse a few more times. Finally, add the flax egg and pulse until the mixture is well combined. Be careful not to overprocess.

✳ PREHEAT THE OVEN to 400°F. Line two rimmed baking sheets with parchment paper. Scoop about ⅓ cup of the mixture in your wet hands and form a ball. Place the ball on the parchment paper and form into a ½-inch-thick round patty. Repeat with the rest of the mixture. (If too moist, place the mixture in the freezer for 5 minutes.)

✳ PLACE THE BAKING SHEETS in the oven. Remove after 15 minutes and flip the patties carefully with a spatula. Return them to the oven and bake for another 10 to 15 minutes, until the burgers are golden brown. Remove the baking sheets from the oven. Let the patties cool for 5 minutes before serving. Store leftover patties in an airtight container in the refrigerator for up to 4 days or in the freezer for 1 month.

NOTE: The patties can be reheated in a toaster oven.

Vegetable Stir-Fry (with Shrimp)

Stir-fry dishes are great to make in the middle of the week when you want to throw together a healthy meal but are short on time. The beauty of stir-fry dishes is that you can just open up the vegetable drawer and use what you have on hand.

*SERVES 2 TO 4

Ingredients

1 tablespoon coconut oil or olive oil

1 small red onion, sliced

1 head of broccoli, cut into bite-size florets

1 cup sliced mushrooms

1 red or orange bell pepper, cored, seeded, and sliced into
  small strips

½ cup snow peas, ends removed

2 carrots, sliced into thin rounds

2 cloves garlic, minced

MARINADE

½-inch piece of fresh ginger, grated

1 tablespoon tamari

1 tablespoon water

½ teaspoon mirin

1 teaspoon maple syrup

1 teaspoon red pepper flakes

1 tablespoon freshly squeezed orange juice

Method

✻ HEAT A SAUTÉ PAN over medium heat. Add the coconut oil and onion. Sauté the onion for 2 minutes. Add the broccoli, mushrooms, bell pepper, snow peas, carrot, and garlic to the pan. Cook for another 3 minutes. To make the marinade, mix the ginger, tamari, water, mirin, maple syrup, red pepper flakes, and orange juice in a small bowl. Whisk together. Allow the marinade to condense for 2 to 3 minutes. Pour the marinade over the vegetables. Serve with brown rice or on its own.

OPTIONAL: Add ½ pound of peeled and deveined small to medium shrimp at the same time that the marinade is added. Cook for 3 to 4 minutes, or until the shrimp curl and turn light pink.

Broiled Miso Orange Glazed Salmon

Salmon is rich in protein, omega-3 fatty acids, and vitamin D. The combination of sweet and salty in the miso-glazed marinade takes it to the next level on taste and flavor. Serve this dish right out of the oven over sautéed greens, or use in a bowl or salad the next day.

*SERVES 2

Ingredients

MARINADE

1 tablespoon white miso

1 tablespoon freshly squeezed orange juice

1 teaspoon minced fresh ginger

1 teaspoon maple syrup or raw honey

1 to 2 teaspoons tamari

½ teaspoon toasted sesame oil

½ teaspoon red pepper flakes

Two 6-ounce salmon fillets

Method

✳ PREHEAT THE BROILER to 500°F. In a small bowl, make the marinade: mix the miso, orange juice, ginger, maple syrup, tamari, sesame oil, and red pepper flakes together. Place the salmon fillets skin-side down in a baking dish. Cover with the marinade. Set aside for at least 30 minutes. Place the marinated salmon in the oven (at least 6 inches from the top), and cook for 6 to 8 minutes for medium-rare doneness. Serve over mixed greens, quinoa, or brown rice.

NOTE: The salmon can also be made on the grill.

Chili Lime Chicken with Fruit Salsa

This chicken is easy to make and flavorful. It's also a total crowd-pleaser and popular with adults and kids alike. Serve in strips with the phytonutrient-rich and colorful Fruit Salsa.

*SERVES 4

Ingredients

Freshly squeezed juice of 2 limes

1 tablespoon olive oil

1 tablespoon raw honey

1 large clove garlic, minced

1½ teaspoons chili powder

½ teaspoon sea salt

4 boneless, skinless chicken breast halves

Fruit Salsa (recipe follows)

Method

✳ IN A MEDIUM BOWL, whisk together the lime juice, olive oil, honey, garlic, chili powder, and salt. Pour the marinade into a shallow dish. Add the chicken breasts and toss well to coat. Chill for 4 hours or overnight, turning at least once.

Heat the grill to medium-high. Remove the chicken from the marinade; discard any excess juices. Grill the chicken approximately 12 minutes, or until it reaches an internal temperature of 170°F, turning once. Transfer the chicken to a platter; let stand 5 to 10 minutes before slicing into strips. Serve with Fruit Salsa.

Fruit Salsa

Ingredients

    8 strawberries, diced
    ½ avocado, pitted and diced
    ½ large mango, pitted and cubed
    ½ small white onion, diced (about ⅓ cup)
    1 tablespoon finely chopped fresh cilantro
    Freshly squeezed juice of 1 lime
    ½ teaspoon chili powder
    Sea salt to taste

Method

IN A SMALL BOWL, toss together the chopped strawberries, avocado, mango, onion, cilantro, lime juice, and chili powder. Season with salt to taste.

VARIATION: Use 1 whole mango and omit the strawberries, or try 4 peaches in place of the mango and strawberries.

Honey Roasted Chicken

This simple chicken dish is perfect for those nights when the weather just won't cooperate and grilling outdoors is out of the question. Serve with brown rice or the Quinoa with Dried Fruits & Nuts (page 242) for an easy-to-prepare main course.

*SERVES 4

Ingredients

    4 chicken breasts, with ribs
    Sea salt and freshly ground black pepper to taste
    ¼ cup raw honey

2 tablespoons tamari

1 tablespoon Dijon mustard

2 tablespoons olive oil

2 cloves garlic, minced

1 shallot, minced

1 tablespoon fresh rosemary, minced

Method

✳ PREHEAT THE OVEN to 375°F. Arrange the chicken in a baking dish in a single layer. Season with salt and pepper. Combine the honey, tamari, mustard, olive oil, garlic, and shallot in the bowl of a food processor, or blend with an immersion blender. Brush the mixture on the chicken. Roast the chicken in the oven for 15 minutes. Remove it from the oven and baste with additional sauce. Roast for 15 minutes more, or until the chicken breasts reach an internal temperature of 170°F. Garnish with rosemary and serve immediately.

Roasted Chicken with Vegetables

With chopped carrots, sweet potatoes, onion, and celery, this is a one-pan dish that includes an array of Live Dirty, Eat Clean players. As the vegetables caramelize, the lemon seeps in and seals in the natural juices of the chicken.

*SERVES 4

Ingredients

1 free-range roasting chicken (approximately 6 pounds)

1 lemon

1 large onion, peeled and sliced in half

2 or 3 fresh sprigs rosemary, plus more sprigs for garnish

Kosher salt and freshly ground black pepper to taste

Fresh poultry seasoning

3 carrots, sliced in thick rounds

2 medium sweet potatoes, chopped

3 stalks celery, sliced into 2-inch pieces

3 cloves garlic

Olive oil

½ cup organic chicken broth

Method

✳ PREHEAT THE OVEN to 450°F. Rinse the chicken, pat it dry, and remove the giblets. Cut the lemon in half and squeeze lemon juice on the chicken skin. Place the onion and the rosemary sprigs in the chicken cavity. Season the cavity with salt and pepper. Generously season the chicken all over with salt, pepper, and fresh poultry seasoning. Place the chicken in a roasting pan.

✳ IN A LARGE BOWL, mix the carrots, sweet potatoes, celery, and garlic. Lightly cover with olive oil and season with salt and pepper. Arrange the vegetables around the chicken.

✳ PLACE THE ROASTING PAN on a rack. Pour the broth over the chicken and roast in the oven for 30 minutes. Stir the vegetables once during the cooking time. Reduce the heat to 375°F and continue to roast for at least an hour more, until the juices run clear and the internal temperature reaches 170°F. Remove the chicken from the oven and let stand for about 5 minutes. Garnish with fresh herb sprigs.

Turkey Burgers

These Asian-inspired burgers are full of intense flavor and contain beneficial microbiome ingredients such as garlic and onion. Whip these up for dinner over a bed of greens or in a lettuce cup. Add a serving of brown rice for a more filling meal. Make sure to keep some extras on hand to toss into a salad or bowl the next day.

*SERVES 4 TO 6

Ingredients

1 pound ground turkey breast

3 teaspoons finely grated fresh ginger root

2 cloves garlic, chopped

1 large egg

1 large carrot, finely grated

2 tablespoons tamari

2 teaspoons sesame oil

1 tablespoon minced fresh cilantro (optional)

3 green onions, minced

Salt and freshly ground black pepper to taste

Olive oil for the griddle

Method

✳ IN A MEDIUM BOWL, combine the turkey, ginger, garlic, egg, carrot, tamari, sesame oil, cilantro, green onions, salt, and pepper. Form the mixture into patties 1½ to 2 inches in diameter. Place the patties on a lightly oiled griddle or pan over medium-high heat for about 7 minutes per side, or until cooked through.

Flank Steak

This dish is adult- and kid-friendly and can be served to a crowd. It pairs perfectly with plain brown rice and green veggies or can be tossed into an Asian-inspired salad the next day.

*SERVES 6

Ingredients

2 cloves garlic, minced

1 tablespoon grated fresh ginger

2 green onions, sliced

½ cup tamari

2 tablespoons olive oil

1 tablespoon sesame oil

2 tablespoons raw honey

1 flank steak (about 1½ pounds)

Method

✳ TO MAKE THE MARINADE, whisk the garlic, ginger, green onions, tamari, olive oil, sesame oil, and honey together in a small bowl. Place the steak in a shallow nonaluminum dish. Pour the marinade over the steak. Turn to coat and marinate the steak for at least 4 hours but preferably overnight. Cook the steak on a grill until medium. Let it rest for a few minutes to seal in the flavors. Cut the steak into thin diagonal slices against the grain of the meat.

Green Bananas

These are a favorite Live Dirty, Eat Clean starch—good for your microbes, your waistline, and your blood sugar. Pair them with veggies or animal protein for a delicious meal.

*SERVES 2 TO 4

Ingredients

   3 unripened green bananas
   2 tablespoons clarified butter or ghee (optional)
   Sea salt and freshly ground black pepper to taste

Method

✳ PLACE THE UNPEELED green bananas in a medium pot and fill with enough water to cover them by an inch. You may need to cut them in half to fit in the pot. Bring the water to a boil over high heat and cook uncovered for 15 to 20 minutes. When they're done, they should feel tender when you poke them with a fork, and the skins may turn dark brown or black with cooking. Remove the bananas from the water and allow them to cool slightly. Remove the skins and mash the green bananas with a fork, adding in the clarified butter if desired. Season with salt and pepper to taste. These are great with Vegetable Stir-Fry (with Shrimp) (page 233), Flank Steak (page 239), Turkey Burgers (page 238), Broiled Miso Orange Glazed Salmon (page 234), or any of the chicken dishes.

Curry & Turmeric Roasted Cauliflower

While cauliflower is pretty bland on its own, the addition of curry and turmeric gives this dish deep flavor along with some microbial health benefits. Roast a batch at the beginning of the week and serve hot, and save any remaining florets to use in salads or bowls over the next few days.

*SERVES 2 TO 4

Ingredients

> 1 head cauliflower, cut into bite-size florets
>
> 1 tablespoon curry powder
>
> 1 teaspoon ground turmeric (or 1 tablespoon fresh turmeric)
>
> 2 tablespoons olive oil
>
> Sea salt and freshly ground black pepper to taste

Method

✳ PREHEAT THE OVEN to 400°F. Lightly oil a roasting pan or rimmed sheet pan. In a large mixing bowl, toss cauliflower with the curry powder, turmeric, olive oil, salt, and pepper. Place on the pan. Roast for 20 to 25 minutes, until the edges of the florets are slightly brown.

Cauliflower Mash with Garlic

Who doesn't love a heaping scoop of "mashed potatoes" to complement dinner? Loaded with nutrients and flavor, this cauliflower version will fill you up without filling you out.

*SERVES 4 TO 6

Ingredients

> 1 head cauliflower, cut into small florets
>
> 2 tablespoons olive oil, clarified butter, or ghee, plus a drizzle to
>> cook the garlic
>
> 1 clove garlic, minced
>
> Splash of unsweetened plant-based milk (optional; for a creamier
>> consistency)
>
> Salt and freshly ground black pepper to taste
>
> 1 tablespoon fresh chives or green onion, sliced and reserved for
>> garnish

Method

✳ BRING A LARGE POT of salted water to a boil over high heat. Add the cauliflower and reduce the heat to a simmer. Cover and cook the cauliflower for about 10 minutes, or until tender. While the cauliflower is cooking, drizzle a drop of olive oil in a small pan over medium heat and cook the garlic until softened and slightly browned, about 2 minutes. Remove from the heat.

✳ DRAIN THE COOKED CAULIFLOWER and place it in a medium bowl. Transfer half of the cauliflower to the bowl of a food processor or high-speed blender; cover and puree until smooth. Add the remaining cauliflower in small batches and puree until the vegetables are smooth and creamy. Blend in the 2 tablespoons of olive oil and the garlic. (Optional: Add a splash of almond milk for a creamier consistency.) Season with salt and pepper to taste. Garnish with the chives.

Quinoa with Dried Fruits & Nuts

This flavorful and colorful quinoa dish is an excellent source of plant-based protein and fiber that can be served on its own or alongside fish and chicken. The combination of vegetables, dried fruits, and nuts makes this a microbiome winner that you will want to serve over and over again.

*SERVES 8

Ingredients

1 cup raw quinoa

2 cups water

Sea salt to taste

1 clove garlic, chopped

Zest of 2 limes

2 to 3 tablespoons freshly squeezed lime juice

2 tablespoons finely chopped green onion

½ jalapeño pepper, seeded and finely chopped

½ teaspoon cumin seeds

½ teaspoon coriander seeds

¼ teaspoon dry mustard

⅓ cup olive oil

8 dried apricots, finely chopped

½ cup dried cherries or cranberries

3 tablespoons finely chopped fresh parsley

1 red, yellow, or orange bell pepper, finely chopped

½ cup toasted pine nuts

Method

✴ RINSE THE QUINOA in a bowl of cold water. Bring the 2 cups water for the quinoa to a boil over medium-high heat in a small saucepan. Season the water with salt. Add the quinoa, reduce the heat to low, cover the pan, and simmer for 15 minutes. Let the quinoa stand for 30 minutes or until cooled.

✴ WHILE THE QUINOA is cooling, make the salad dressing: combine the garlic, lime zest, lime juice, green onion, jalapeño, cumin, coriander, and dry mustard in a large bowl. Next, slowly whisk in the olive oil to form an emulsion. Toss the cooked quinoa with ¼ cup of the dressing.

✴ ADD THE DRIED FRUITS, parsley, bell pepper, and pine nuts to the quinoa. Add enough of remaining dressing to coat the mixture. Season with salt to taste. Serve as a side dish or use it as a bed for an entrée.

Roasted Brussels Sprouts

Brussels sprouts are an excellent source of indigestible plant fiber. Add them as a side to any main dish, and don't forget to make extras to toss into a bowl (see page 226) or salad the next day.

*SERVES 6

Ingredients

1½ pounds Brussels sprouts

1 to 2 tablespoons olive oil (enough to coat)

Kosher salt to taste

½ teaspoon freshly ground black pepper

Method

✴ PREHEAT THE OVEN to 400°F. Cut off the ends of the Brussels sprouts and pull off any brown outer leaves. Slice them in half lengthwise. Mix the Brussels sprouts in a bowl with the olive oil, salt, and pepper. Place the vegetables on a rimmed baking sheet and roast for 30 to 35 minutes. Stir the Brussels sprouts occasionally to brown them evenly. The Brussels sprouts are done when they are crispy on the outside and tender on the inside.

Roasted Fennel

Even if you're not a fan of the licorice taste in raw fennel, give this recipe a try. Roasting fennel brings out a nutty sweetness. Serve alongside any of the mains or toss it into a bowl of quinoa or brown rice.

*SERVES 2

Ingredients

2 bulbs fennel

3 tablespoons olive oil

Sea salt and freshly ground black pepper to taste

1 tablespoon of any combination of rosemary, thyme, and
    basil (optional)

Method

❋ PREHEAT THE OVEN to 400°F. Remove the stems of the fennel, slice the bulbs in half lengthwise, then slice vertically into ½-inch pieces. Coat the fennel with the olive oil, salt, pepper, and herbs if using. Place the fennel on a parchment-lined rimmed baking sheet. Roast for 20 minutes and then stir the fennel. Bake for 15 to 20 minutes more, until the edges are slightly browned and crisp.

Roasted Asparagus

This simple roasted recipe is a surefire, tasty way to get your green on and fill your plate with microbe-boosting inulin fiber.

*SERVES 4

Ingredients

1 bunch asparagus

½ to 1 teaspoon minced fresh garlic

Salt and freshly ground black pepper to taste

2 tablespoons olive oil (or enough to coat)

½ lemon

Method

✳ PREHEAT THE OVEN to 400°F. Place the asparagus, garlic, salt, pepper, and olive oil in a bowl. Toss to coat. Spread the asparagus on a rimmed baking sheet in a single layer. Roast for 12 to 16 minutes, or until tender but still crisp. Turn only once during the cooking time. Lightly squeeze the lemon over the spears just before serving.

Baked Root Vegetable Chips

Root veggies such as carrots, parsnips, beets, yams, sweet potatoes, rutabagas, turnips, onions, and even ginger grow underneath the ground where they're not only the anchor and foundation of a plant, but they also soak in enormous amounts of minerals. Bonus: When you roast or bake root vegetables, they caramelize into a glorious sweet flavor, perfect for curbing sweet cravings. Serve these on their own or as a crunchy side with soup or salad.

Ingredients

Mix and match any of these root veggies: golden beets, red beets, sweet potatoes, parsnips, rutabagas, turnips

Olive oil (enough to lightly oil the tray and vegetables)

Sea salt to taste

OPTIONAL: Add herbs and spices for variety. Try parsley, rosemary, garlic granules, chili powder, cumin, or paprika.

Method

✳ PREHEAT THE OVEN to 400°F. Peel the vegetables and slice them into about ⅛-inch-thick rounds using a mandolin, handheld slicer, or knife. In a large bowl filled with cold water, soak the sliced vegetables for about 10 minutes. (This step is not mandatory, but it will help them get crispy. Soak beets in a separate bowl to avoid turning the other veggies pink.) Pat each slice dry.

✳ NEXT, use 2 or 3 rimmed baking sheets and brush each with a thin layer of olive oil. Place the veggie slices on the lightly oiled baking sheets, making sure they don't overlap. Then brush each slice with olive oil and sprinkle with salt.

(You will likely need to roast the veggie chips in a few batches.) Place the baking sheets in the oven and bake for 20 to 25 minutes, flipping about halfway through. For the last 10 minutes, check frequently to avoid burning. Remove the smaller chips first, once the edges are crispy and the chips are starting to curl up.

✳ THE CHIPS SHOULD CRISP UP even more once cooled. Sprinkle with additional salt and seasonings, if using, to taste.

NOTE: These are best eaten right away.

Bring on More Root Veggies

Instead of baked chips, turn on the oven and roast your roots in chunks or slice them into thin strips to make sweet potato, parsnip, or carrot fries. You can also toss any leftovers into a salad the next day (see Roasted Root Vegetable Salad, page 220).

SOUPS & BROTHS

Vibrant Veggie Soup

This fiber-filled and colorful soup is a great way to get in your veggies. It's a Live Dirty, Eat Clean Lifestyle staple to enjoy for lunch alongside a salad, in the afternoon as a warming snack, or as an appetizer before dinner to take the edge off your hunger. This soup is very versatile and can be adapted with different vegetables, depending on the season and availability.

*SERVES 8 TO 10

Ingredients

  2 tablespoons high-quality olive oil

  1 yellow or sweet onion, diced

  2 cloves garlic, chopped

  3 stalks celery, chopped

  4 carrots, chopped

2 tablespoons chopped fresh herbs (parsley, oregano, and/or thyme)

4 cups vegetable broth

1½ cups cooked white beans

3 cups fresh tomatoes, chopped, with juices

6 ounces tomato paste* (preferably from a glass jar or tube, not a can)

6 cups chopped vegetables (broccoli, red bell pepper, yellow
     squash, zucchini, green beans, mushrooms, cauliflower, etc.)

1 to 2 cups water, depending on desired consistency (can use broth
     instead)

3 cups fresh spinach leaves (reserve until the end)

Sea salt and freshly ground black pepper to taste

Red pepper flakes (optional; for an additional kick)

*Due to the acid in the tomatoes and the possibility of BPA in cans, choose fresh first, then a tube or glass over canned when possible.

Method

✳ HEAT THE OLIVE OIL in a stockpot over medium heat and add the onion, garlic, celery, and carrot. Sauté until the onion is lightly browned, then add the fresh herbs to coat vegetables. Next, add the broth, white beans, tomatoes, and tomato paste. Mix thoroughly and then place the chopped vegetables in the pot. Add enough water to cover the vegetables. Bring to a boil, reduce the heat to a simmer, cover, and cook for about 40 minutes. When the veggies are soft, remove the pot from the heat and add in the spinach leaves. Cover the pot for 5 minutes to allow the spinach to steam. Season with salt and fresh pepper. Add in red pepper flakes, if desired.

Chicken & Veggie Immunity Soup

Whip up a batch of this soup when you need a boost. With the healing spices—garlic, ginger, and turmeric—it's hard not to feel better after one bowl of this nourishing soup. For a denser soup, add in a serving of quinoa or brown rice.

*SERVES 6 TO 8

Ingredients

    1 pound skinless, boneless chicken breast, cut into 1-inch chunks

    2 tablespoons olive oil or coconut oil

    1 onion, diced

    1 to 2 cloves garlic, minced

    1 tablespoon freshly grated ginger

    1½ tablespoons freshly grated turmeric

    4 carrots, thinly sliced

    2 stalks celery, thinly sliced

    ¼ cup coarsely chopped fresh parsley

    1 zucchini, diced

    1 yellow squash, diced

    4 cups chicken broth

    1 cup filtered water

    2 cups spinach

    1 lemon

    1 teaspoon sea salt, plus more to taste

    Freshly ground black pepper to taste

    Red pepper flakes (optional)

Method

✻ CUT THE CHICKEN BREAST into 1-inch cubes. In a large stockpot, heat the olive oil over medium-high heat and add the chicken, onion, and garlic. Sauté for 4 to 5 minutes. Add the ginger and turmeric and stir to coat the chicken with the spices. Cook for 3 to 4 minutes more. Add the carrots and celery and sauté for 2 to 3 minutes. Next, add the parsley, zucchini, and squash to the pan and stir. Add the broth and filtered water. Bring to a boil, cover, and reduce the heat to a simmer. Continue cooking for 30 minutes more. Remove the pot from the heat and add the spinach. Cover for a few minutes to allow the spinach to wilt. Squeeze the juice from the lemon into the soup. Season with salt and pepper to taste. Add in red pepper flakes, if desired.

NOTE: For a meatless option, use cubed butternut squash instead of chicken and vegetable broth instead of chicken broth.

Roasted Butternut Squash Soup

This fall favorite is simple and easy to make and bursting with flavor. The savory roasted vegetables and herbs combine beautifully to create a smooth, creamy, and nourishing soup. Serve garnished with toasted pumpkin seeds and red pepper flakes for a little extra kick.

*SERVES 8

Ingredients

4 cups peeled and coarsely chopped butternut squash

2 cups peeled and coarsely chopped sweet potatoes

3 tablespoons olive oil

2 large cloves garlic, minced

Sea salt and freshly ground black pepper to taste

1 tablespoon chopped fresh sage (or 1 teaspoon ground)

1 tablespoon chopped fresh thyme

1 large onion, coarsely chopped

2 large carrots, coarsely chopped

2 red bell peppers, coarsely chopped

4 cups vegetable broth, plus more to adjust the consistency of the soup

½ teaspoon red pepper flakes and pumpkin seeds, for garnish

Method

✳ PREHEAT THE OVEN to 375°F. Place the squash and sweet potatoes on two rimmed baking sheets and toss with the olive oil, garlic, salt, pepper, sage, and thyme. Roast for 30 minutes. Remove the baking sheets from the oven, adjust the seasonings, and add the onion, carrots, and bell peppers. Return the baking sheets to the oven and cook for an additional 20 minutes, or until the vegetables are starting to turn a golden brown. Remove baking sheets from the oven and place the roasted vegetables and broth in a large stockpot. Heat over medium-high heat until boiling and then reduce the heat to a simmer. Cook for 20 minutes, or until the vegetables are soft. Once the soup has cooled down a bit, use an immersion blender to puree the soup to a smooth consistency. Add extra broth for a slightly thinner soup. Season with salt and black pepper. Serve in bowls and garnish with red pepper flakes and pumpkin seeds.

NOTE: If an immersion blender is not available, use a food processor or high-speed blender after allowing the soup to cool slightly.

Split Pea Soup/Dal

Split peas are a member of the legume family and are a great source of fiber that can help to grow your gut garden. This versatile dish can be made as a liquid for soup, or a thicker consistency for dal, which can be served over rice or quinoa.

*SERVES 8

Ingredients

1 pound yellow split peas, rinsed and drained

8 to 12 cups low-sodium chicken or vegetable broth, depending on the
desired consistency

4 large cloves garlic, minced

1 medium yellow onion, minced

2 cups coconut milk (optional)

3 scallions, chopped

1 jalapeño pepper, seeded and diced

1 sprig of fresh thyme

½ teaspoon ground cumin

Freshly ground black pepper to taste

Method

✳ ADD THE SPLIT PEAS and 8 cups broth to a large stockpot, along with the garlic and onion. Bring to a boil over high heat, reduce the heat to medium-high, and cook until the peas are soft, about 1 hour. Add additional broth as needed to keep the mixture liquid. Add the coconut milk if using and boil for 10 minutes. Add the scallions, jalapeño, and thyme and cook for 10 minutes more. Remove the pot from the heat and blend the soup with an immersion blender or puree in a food processor. Return the mixture to medium heat and cook for 30 minutes more. Season with cumin and pepper to taste.

Lentil Soup with Leeks

With resistant starches from the green lentils and inulin from both the leeks and garlic, this recipe has the Live Dirty, Eat Clean name all over it. Make a batch of this nourishing soup over the weekend, and enjoy a few hearty meals throughout the week. Freeze any leftovers in individual containers to pull out in a pinch.

*SERVES 10

Ingredients

3 tablespoons olive oil

2 medium leeks, chopped (white parts only)

1 tablespoon minced garlic

1 tablespoon chopped fresh oregano (or 1 teaspoon dried)

1 teaspoon ground cumin

4 carrots, sliced in rounds

4 stalks celery, thinly sliced

8 cups vegetable broth

2 cups French green lentils, rinsed

½ cup tomato paste

3 cups spinach (reserve until end)

½ lemon

Sea salt and freshly group black pepper to taste

Method

✳ HEAT THE OLIVE OIL in a large pan or Dutch oven over medium heat. Add the leeks, garlic, oregano, and cumin. Cook until the vegetables are soft, 4 to 5 minutes. Next, add the carrots and celery and sauté for an additional 8 minutes. Add the broth, lentils, and tomato paste to the pot and bring to a boil. Reduce the heat to a low simmer and cook for 60 to 70 minutes. The soup is done when the lentils are soft. Remove the pot from the heat and add the spinach. Cover the pot for an additional 5 minutes to wilt the spinach. Squeeze the juice from the half lemon into the soup and stir. Season with salt and pepper to taste.

Easy Gazpacho with Avocado

When it's warm outside, cold and refreshing gazpacho hits the spot. This is one of those dishes that taste better the next day, once all the crisp flavors from the fresh vegetables settle in together. Top with avocado and serve this summer staple in a bowl, or fill up a shot glass for each guest to enjoy at your next dinner party.

*SERVES 6

Ingredients

1 large English cucumber, unpeeled and coarsely chopped

½ small sweet onion, sliced into chunks

2 cloves garlic, peeled

4 to 5 large tomatoes, cored and cut in half

1 tablespoon freshly squeezed lime juice

1 tablespoon sherry vinegar

2 tablespoons olive oil

1 to 2 teaspoons sea salt

Freshly ground black pepper to taste

½ teaspoon red pepper flakes (or more depending on desired spiciness)

1 avocado, peeled and cubed

Method

✳ PLACE THE CUCUMBER into the bowl of a food processor and pulse until coarsely chopped. Transfer it to a separate bowl. Next, repeat the process with the sweet onion and garlic. Add the onion mixture to the cucumber. Place half of the tomatoes in the bowl of the food processor and pulse until the texture is coarse and chunky. Add the chopped tomatoes to the cucumber and onion mixture. Next, process remaining tomatoes, lime juice, vinegar, olive oil, salt, black pepper, and red pepper flakes. Mix until smooth. Place the ingredients in the bowl with the cucumber, onion, and tomato. Stir the mixture, cover, and store in the refrigerator for at least 4 hours or overnight. Once completely chilled, serve with cubed avocado on top.

Homemade Vegetable Broth

A homemade vegetable broth is a must for the Live Dirty, Eat Clean Lifestyle. It can be used to sip on in between meals, as the base of a soup, or instead of water when cooking quinoa and brown rice. Using homemade broth in place of store-bought broth provides a big nutritional boost to all of your dishes. It's also easy to make and doesn't really require measuring. Plus, it's a great way to make sure that all of the veggies you forgot to eat during the week don't get thrown away. Start with this basic guideline, which highlights the microbiome-friendly foods but, like most of the recipes you will find here, you can adjust according to taste and availability.

*MAKES ABOUT 10 CUPS

Ingredients (More or Less)

1 to 2 onions

6 carrots

6 stalks celery

2 cloves garlic, halved

1 to 2 bay leaves

½ bunch fresh flat-leaf parsley

1 to 2 parsnips

1 to 2 leeks

1 fennel bulb

8 to 10 black peppercorns

Sea salt to taste

Approximately 1 gallon cold water (make sure all vegetables are covered)

You can also add: tamari, sweet potatoes, bell peppers, greens, turnips, zucchini, tomatoes, broccoli, kombu (seaweed for minerals), or any vegetable scraps you have

Method

✳ RINSE ALL OF THE vegetables and place in a large stockpot. Cover with water so that the vegetables are completely immersed. Bring to a boil over high heat. Reduce the heat to a simmer and cook uncovered for a minimum of 2 hours. Check to make sure that the vegetables are covered. Add more water if it evaporates too fast. Once the vegetables have cooked completely, strain the broth into a glass bowl. Add salt or a dash of tamari to taste. Once cooled, store in the refrigerator for up to 5 days or freeze in individual containers for up to 4 months.

Bone Broth

Bone broth is another healing food that can be easily integrated into the Live Dirty, Eat Clean Plan. Just like the Homemade Vegetable Broth (page 253), it can be enjoyed on its own or used to add flavor and nutrients to soups, meat dishes, or vegetable and grain dishes. Preparing bone broth is easy and forgiving. Just be sure that you use bones from grass-fed or organic animals. Always use an acid (apple cider vinegar or lemon) to help break down the minerals from the bone, which are healing for the digestive system. You can use a variety of herbs to change up the flavor, and you also can add in whatever bones you have on hand. Try this basic recipe as a guide, and then create your own version of this ultra-nourishing broth.

Ingredients

Bones from 1 whole free-range or organic chicken

2 tablespoons apple cider vinegar

1 large onion, chopped

1 leek (white part only), chopped

2 cloves garlic, minced

3 carrots, peeled and coarsely chopped

3 stalks celery, coarsely chopped

4 quarts filtered water

Fresh herbs: parsley, marjoram, and thyme work well

8 to 10 whole peppercorns

1 bay leaf

Method

✳ WASH ALL OF THE bones thoroughly. Place the chicken bones, vinegar, onion, leek, garlic, carrots, celery, and water to cover in a large stockpot. Let stand for 30 minutes. Next, bring the pot to a hard boil over high heat. Skim the scum that rises to the top of the pot. Reduce the heat, cover, and simmer for 8 to 24 hours. Check periodically to remove the impurities on top of the soup. Add the fresh herbs, peppercorns, and bay leaf about 30 minutes before the end of cooking. After 30 minutes more, remove the bones and then strain the broth. Once cooled, place the broth in the refrigerator until the fat congeals. Remove the fat with a spoon or skimmer, and then store the broth in the refrigerator up to 3 days or in the freezer for up to 6 months.

SNACKS & SWEETS

High-Fiber Trail Mix

Trail mix makes an easy, on-the-go snack that tastes delicious and can help stabilize blood sugar in between meals. Pack up a mason jar and store it in your desk, make individual serving packets to throw in your bag, or bring it along on your next hike.

*MAKES 3¼ CUPS

Ingredients
½ cup sunflower seeds
1 cup walnuts or almonds
1 cup goji berries
½ cup coconut flakes
¼ cup cacao nibs

Method
* MIX THE SUNFLOWER SEEDS, walnuts, berries, coconut flakes, and cacao nibs together in a bowl and store in an airtight container.

No-Bake Energy Balls

These bite-size snacks are delicious and pack a hefty dose of plant-based protein, fiber, and healthy fats. Whip up a batch at the beginning of the week and store in the refrigerator to have any time you need a pick-me-up.

*MAKES 16 TO 18 BALLS

Ingredients

1 cup cashews

1 packed cup pitted Medjool dates

½ cup unsweetened shredded coconut, plus more to roll in

1 tablespoon raw honey or maple syrup

½ teaspoon pure vanilla extract

Pinch of ground cardamom

½ teaspoon Himalayan sea salt

½ cup dried fruit (optional; goji berries, cranberries, or cherries work well) (see Variation below)

Method

✳ PLACE CASHEWS in a the bowl of a food processor and pulse until crumbly, not completely smooth. Next, add the dates, coconut, honey, vanilla, cardamom, and salt. Process until combined. (It will be sticky.) Using a small spoon, scoop out the mixture and roll into bite-size morsels, forming them with your hands. Roll the balls in additional shredded coconut. Store in the refrigerator up to 3 days or in the freezer up to 1 month.

VARIATION: Add dried fruit to the food processor after the mixture is processed and pulse a few times until incorporated.

Dates with Nut Butter

This isn't really a "recipe," but it is the perfect energizing snack that takes only minutes to make. Just slice open a fresh date, remove the pit, and fill it with almond butter (or any no-sugar-added nut butter). Then sprinkle with raw cacao nibs, shredded coconut, cinnamon, or just enjoy au naturel.

Ingredients

Fresh Medjool dates

Nut butter (almond, cashew, peanut, sunflower, or any no-sugar-added variety)

Toppings: raw cacao nibs, shredded coconut, cinnamon

Method

✳ SLICE OPEN THE DATES. Remove the pits. Fill with nut butter. Sprinkle with a topping. Eat immediately.

Chickpea Herbed Crackers

The hardest part of the Live Dirty, Eat Clean Plan for some people is giving up their beloved bread. Fear not! These gluten-free but tasty flatbread-style crackers are the perfect complement to soups, salads, hummus, frittatas, and more.

Ingredients

1 tablespoon flax meal

3 tablespoons cool water, plus ¾ cup warm water

½ cup chickpea flour

1 cup almond flour

½ cup brown rice flour

2 tablespoons olive oil

1½ teaspoons sea salt

2 tablespoons sesame seeds

¼ teaspoon ground turmeric

¼ cup fresh flat-leaf parsley, chopped

1 tablespoon chopped chives

1 tablespoon raw honey

Method

✳ PREHEAT THE OVEN to 325°F. Line a baking pan with parchment paper.

✳ IN A SMALL BOWL, mix the flax meal with the 3 tablespoons of cool water. Let the mixture stand for 10 minutes until a gel-like consistency forms. This makes a flax "egg."

✳ IN THE BOWL of a food processor, combine flax "egg," flours, olive oil, and 1 teaspoon salt. Pulse 10 times. Add in 1 tablespoon of the sesame seeds, the turmeric, parsley, chives, and raw honey and pulse until combined. With the processor running, slowly pour in the ¾ cup warm water and process until the dough comes together. The mixture should resemble a thick batter. Spread evenly on the parchment-lined baking sheet with a spatula until the dough is paper thin. Sprinkle the remaining 1 tablespoon of sesame seeds and additional ½ teaspoon of sea salt on top. Bake for 25 minutes, or until the edges become firm and the crackers are golden brown. Remove the tray from the oven and allow to cool before breaking into bite-size pieces. The crackers can be kept for up to 4 days in an airtight container. Toast before serving, for optimal crispiness.

Seeded Almond Flour Bread

This homemade gluten-free and grain-free loaf is made with almond flour. It has a nice, dense texture that pairs perfectly with sliced avocado for "avo toast," or it can be enjoyed with some Raspberry Chia Seed Jam (page 259) and a little nut butter for a healthy PB&J.

*MAKES ONE LOAF (ABOUT 12 SLICES)

Ingredients

Olive oil or coconut oil for greasing the loaf pan

2½ cups almond flour

½ teaspoon baking soda

½ teaspoon sea salt

3 large eggs

1 tablespoon maple syrup or raw honey

1 teaspoon apple cider vinegar

2 tablespoons mixed seeds (pumpkin and sunflower seeds work best)

Method

✳ PREHEAT THE OVEN to 300°F. Use a small amount of olive oil to grease a 9 x 5-inch loaf pan. In a medium bowl, mix together the almond flour, baking soda, and salt. In a separate small bowl, whisk the eggs, the maple syrup, and vinegar together. Once blended, add the egg mixture to the dry ingredients. Pour the mixture into the prepared loaf pan and sprinkle the seeds on top. Bake for about 45 minutes. The loaf should be golden on top and brown around the edges when it's done.

Raspberry Chia Seed Jam

Here's a jam that doesn't require any canning experience and can be made in only a matter of minutes. Start with the raspberry flavor, then experiment with other berries or a mixture of them all. Serve on the Seeded Almond Flour Bread (page 258), mixed into oatmeal, or as a sweet layer in a coconut yogurt parfait.

*SERVES 6 TO 8

Ingredients

1½ cups raspberries (can use fresh or thawed frozen)

¼ cup water (use only for fresh berries)

1 to 2 tablespoons maple syrup

½ teaspoon lemon zest

2 tablespoons chia seeds

Method

✴ IN A BOWL, mash the berries with a fork. (Add the water if using fresh berries.) Place the mashed berries, maple syrup, and lemon zest in a small pot. Bring to a boil over high heat, then reduce the heat to a simmer. Stir for 3 to 4 minutes. Remove the pot from the heat and mix in the chia seeds. Once cooled, place the thickened mixture in a mason jar or airtight container and store in the refrigerator for up to 2 weeks.

Guilt-Free Chocolate Orange Truffles

Aside from being delicious bite-size treats, these easy, no-bake truffles are filled with nourishing ingredients that aren't present in the commercial varieties. Be prepared to get a little messy before enjoying every morsel of this decadent but guilt-free dessert.

*MAKES 18 TO 20 TRUFFLES

Ingredients

1 cup cashews or almonds

¾ cup packed Medjool dates, pitted

¼ cup unsweetened cocoa powder or raw cacao powder

Pinch of sea salt

1 teaspoon pure vanilla extract

1 tablespoon orange zest

Unsweetened cocoa powder or raw cacao powder for dusting

Method

✳ PLACE THE CASHEWS in the bowl of a food processor and blend until finely ground. Add in the dates, cocoa powder, salt, and vanilla. Once the mixture is smooth, pulse in the orange zest and process until everything is incorporated together. Next, with slightly wet hands, roll the mixture into 1-inch balls. (If the mixture is too sticky to handle, place in the freezer for 15 to 20 minutes, until firm enough to roll.) Lightly cover each truffle with cocoa powder. Place them in the refrigerator for at least an hour before serving. Store any remaining truffles in an airtight glass container for up to 3 days in the refrigerator or freeze to have on hand always.

Chocolate Mousse

This healthy yet decadent chocolate mousse tastes like the "real deal" with each creamy and rich spoonful. Enjoying pleasurable but healthy foods, including dessert, is a big part of the Live Dirty, Eat Clean Diet. So, go ahead . . . you're in for a nutrient-dense treat.

*SERVES 2

Ingredients

1 ripe avocado, pitted and peeled

¼ cup unsweetened cocoa powder or raw cacao powder

¼ cup coconut or almond milk (start with less and adjust to desired consistency)

3 tablespoons maple syrup

1 teaspoon pure vanilla extract

Pinch of sea salt

Optional toppings: shredded coconut, fresh berries, banana slices, cacao nibs, sprinkle of cinnamon

Method

✳ PLACE THE AVOCADO, cocoa powder, coconut milk, maple syrup, vanilla, and salt in the bowl of a food processor or high-speed blender. Slowly add in a splash or two of coconut milk, until the mixture reaches the desired consistency. (This is a thick dessert.) Place the mousse in the refrigerator for at least an hour to let the flavors set before serving. Store in the refrigerator for up to 2 days. Serve in individual small bowls and top with shredded coconut and fresh berries or other optional toppings.

Grain-Free Chocolate Chip Cookies

These are my favorite cookies. With almond flour and just a touch of honey and molasses, you can satisfy your sweet tooth without wreaking havoc on your microbiome.

*MAKES 12 COOKIES

Ingredients

2 cups almond flour

½ teaspoon baking soda

½ teaspoon sea salt

¼ cup organic raw honey

1 teaspoon molasses

1½ teaspoons pure vanilla extract

½ cup organic clarified butter (or substitute coconut oil at room temperature)

¾ cup semisweet chocolate chips

Method

✳ PREHEAT THE OVEN to 350°F. Line a baking sheet with parchment paper. Add the almond flour, baking soda, and salt to the bowl of a food processor and mix well. Add the honey, molasses, vanilla, and clarified butter to the mixture. Process until it becomes a dough. Transfer to a bowl, add the chocolate, and mix. Drop the dough by rounded tablespoons onto the baking sheet at least 2 inches apart. Bake for 7 to 9 minutes, until the tops of the cookies are set and the edges begin to brown. Allow to cool on the pan for 10 minutes before transferring to a wire rack to cool completely. These cookies are best eaten while still warm, but they'll keep for 2 to 3 days in an airtight container or up to 1 month in the freezer.

Live Dirty, Eat Clean "Ice Cream"

Who doesn't love ice cream? You can indulge with this guilt-free, incredibly healthy, easy-to-make, and delicious version. All you need are bananas and a blender or food processor, and you can whip up a batch in no time. Open up a probiotic to sprinkle in, and you'll be doing your microbiome a favor at the same time. Use this simple recipe as a base, and then mix and match for your own customizable flavor.

*SERVES 2

Ingredients

3 ripe bananas, peeled, sliced, and frozen

2 capsules probiotics

VARIATIONS: Add almond butter, peanut butter, blueberries, strawberries, raspberries, mango, cocoa (or raw cacao powder), pureed pumpkin, ginger, cinnamon, vanilla, or mint.

Method

✳ BLEND THE BANANAS in the bowl of a food processor or a high-speed blender. Before the mixture becomes smooth, it will appear chunky. Scrape down the sides. (Add variations at this point, if desired.) Then pulse until the batter achieves a smooth, creamy, soft-serve texture. Place the "ice cream" in a bowl and mix in the probiotic so that it is evenly distributed. Top with fruit, shredded coconut, or nuts or eat plain and simple. Consume immediately (recommended) or store in an airtight glass container in the freezer for up to 1 week.

Mint Chip Dessert Smoothie

If you loved mint chip ice cream as a kid, then you are going to freak out over this nutrient-dense but scrumptious dessert. Who knew that a smoothie thick enough to be soft-serve ice cream that is made with greens from spinach and avocados could remind us of one of our favorite childhood treats?

*SERVES 4

Ingredients

¾ cup unsweetened almond or coconut milk (see DIY Nut Milk, page 213)

4 cups spinach leaves

4 Medjool dates, pitted

8 sprigs of fresh mint leaves (or ½ teaspoon mint extract if fresh mint is not an option)

1 ripe avocado, pitted and peeled

1 teaspoon pure vanilla extract

2 large ripe bananas, frozen and cut into chunks (peel and slice prior to freezing)

2 tablespoons chocolate chips or cacao nibs

Method

✳ PLACE THE PLANT-BASED MILK and spinach in the bowl of a high-speed blender and blend. Next, add the dates and mint leaves and blend. Toss in the avocado, vanilla, and bananas and blend until the mixture is smooth, thick, and creamy. Add ice if necessary. Use a spoon and mix in the chocolate chips, then dish into small bowls.

Fermented Foods

Recipes on pages 263–271: Reprinted from *The Essential Book of Fermentation: Great Taste and Good Health with Probiotic Foods* by arrangement with Avery, a member of Penguin Group (USA) LLC, a Penguin Random House Company, copyright © 2013 by Jeff Cox.

Coconut Milk Kefir

Kefir is a tangy, milk- or water-based drink fermented by a symbiotic combination of bacteria and yeast clumped together in a matrix of pro-

tein, fats, and sugar. It's a wonderfully rich source of healthy, diverse microbes and will do you a world of good. Kefir originated in the North Caucasus region, but no one knows precisely where or when. It comes to us from the mists of time, most likely handed down through many hundreds of generations.

You can buy commercial kefir at the store, but you'll make a better version at home. The symbiotic combination of bacteria and yeast forms "grains" that resemble small cauliflower florets. Some scientific sources have found up to thirty different kinds of bacteria in the grains.

*SERVES 2

Ingredients

½ cup milk kefir grains, unwashed

2 cups coconut milk

Method

✳ PLACE THE KEFIR GRAINS in a widemouthed quart canning jar and pour in the coconut milk. Lay a square of paper towel across the top and screw down the lid band (but not the lid). Allow the coconut milk to culture at room temperature for 12 to 15 hours, less time for warmer temperatures, more time for cooler temperatures, until the milk is cultured and thick. If the first batch fails to culture, pour off the coconut milk and reserve in the refrigerator for other uses, and make a second or third batch if needed. Use a plastic strainer and spoon to retrieve the cultured coconut milk curds as you would for milk kefir, adding the grains back to the quart jar to make tomorrow's batch.

Kimchi

This is the recipe for kimchi that I suggest you start with. You can add and subtract vegetables as you see fit, and as vegetables become available through the seasons. Just be aware that summertime kimchi will ferment rapidly, while cold winter kimchi will take more time to get just right. And remember, too, that refrigeration slows fermentation to a crawl, putting the microbes into a kind of suspended animation. This recipe can be dou-

bled or tripled, depending on how many hungry kimchi recipients are waiting. Of course, all ingredients should be organic. Vegetables or other ingredients dosed with pesticides or preservatives will kill off or set back the beneficial fermentation microbes.

*MAKES 3 OR 4 PINTS

Ingredients

VEGETABLES

½ cup sea salt

2 quarts filtered or spring water

1 large head napa cabbage

3 medium carrots

1 daikon radish

3 scallions

PASTE

3 serrano chilies, or to taste

5-inch piece fresh ginger, peeled and grated

6 cloves garlic, peeled and minced

½ cup fish sauce (without preservatives)

Method

✳ TO MAKE THE VEGETABLES, place the salt and water in a ceramic crock or glass container and stir until dissolved. Remove the outer leaves from the napa cabbage and slice the remainder crosswise into ¼-inch slices. Place these in the crock with the brine. Slice the carrots, daikon radish, and scallions into very thin rounds and mix them into the cabbage and brine. Place a plate on the vegetables to hold them under the brine. Weigh down the plate with a closed jar of liquid, bottle of wine, or gallon-size, closed zip-top freezer bag with at least a quart of water in it for 6 hours, either during the day or overnight. After the soak, drain the vegetables in a colander and place them in a bowl. Reserve the liquid brine. To make the paste, stem the chilies and slice them in half lengthwise. Use as is if you want a hot and spicy kimchi, or for less heat, remove the seeds and membrane and discard. Mince the chilies and place them in a bowl. Add the ginger, garlic, and fish sauce to the bowl with the chilies. Transfer to the bowl of a food processor or blender and whiz to a thick paste. Put half the vegetables and half the paste back into the original crock or jar and mix thoroughly. Add the remaining vegetables and paste and mix thoroughly again. Crush the vegetables with your hands, as if performing deep-tissue massage, squeezing and crushing, for about 5 minutes, until all of the vegetables are thoroughly crunched.

✳ PUT A PLATE ON the vegetables in the crock to push them slightly under the juices. If the top seems dry, add a little of the reserved brine to make sure everything is wet. Put a weight, such as a closed quart jar of water, on top of the plate to keep the vegetables under the surface. Cover the crock containing the submerged ingredients with a cloth to keep out insects. Punch down the kimchi every day for a week to release carbon dioxide gases and to mix the ingredients. When it tastes right, about a week or two later, spoon the kimchi into canning jars, add a little of the brining liquid so everything stays wet, screw on the lids with metal bands, and store in the refrigerator for up to 4 weeks. When you open the jars to use some of the kimchi, you'll allow any buildup of CO_2 to escape. Be sure to share with family and friends.

Garlic Dill Pickles

This recipe can be scaled up or down, but I wanted to give you the basic instructions for 10 pounds of cukes. As for equipment, have a vegetable brush handy. You'll need a 5-gallon ceramic or glass crock or a 5-gallon bucket of food-grade plastic. Please make sure it's food-grade; that is, it originally was used to hold food. Other plastics leach toxic chemicals into their contents. You'll need a glass or ceramic plate that just fits inside the crock or bucket, plus an unused gallon-size zip-top freezer bag, clean dish towels, a fresh package of cheesecloth, a large stainless steel or other nonreactive metal pot, a carton of canning jars with lids and bands, and a narrow plastic spatula.

Note that the recipe calls for pickling spices. You can find them in the spice rack at almost any supermarket, but if you want to make your own, mix together crushed cinnamon sticks; bay leaves; ground allspice, mace, and ginger; the whole seeds of mustard, dill, black peppercorns, coriander, juniper berries, and cardamom; plus whole cloves.

*MAKES 3 OR 4 QUART JARS, DEPENDING ON THE SIZE OF THE CUKES

Ingredients

    10 pounds unwaxed pickling cucumbers

    ¼ cup pickling spices

    2 bunches fresh dill

    1 cup white vinegar

    1 gallon spring or filtered water

    ¾ cup coarse pickling salt (not iodized) or sea salt

    10 cloves garlic, peeled

Method

* SCRUB THE SURFACE OF cucumbers under cool running water to remove any incidental soil. Cut ¹⁄₁₆ inch off the blossom end of the cukes. Blossom ends contain enzymes that can render your pickles soft. Cut the stem ends back to where the cucumber flesh starts. Discard any cukes that are discolored, bruised, or soft. Put half the pickling spices and 1 bunch of dill in the bottom of your fermenting vessel. Add all of the cucumbers. Mix the vinegar and water in a large bowl. Add the pickling salt and stir to dissolve it completely. Pour the mixture over the cucumbers. Add the garlic, the rest of the pickling spices, and the second bunch of dill.

* THE CUCUMBERS MUST BE fully submerged under the brine at all times during the fermentation. Use a glass or ceramic plate that just fits in the vessel to weigh them down. Fill the gallon freezer bag with more vinegar-salt-water brine, zip it tightly, and set it on the plate. Cover the vessel with a clean dish towel and place the crock in a spot where a temperature of from 70°F to 75°F is maintained. *Lactobacilli* work best at this temperature. Lower or higher temperatures favor unwanted spoilage bacteria or fungus spores.

* CHECK THE CROCK EVERY DAY, but don't taste the pickles. After a day or two, you'll see some scum forming on the surface of the brine. This is yeast growth and must be removed or the pickles will spoil. Remove it every day. Keep the brine topped up with extra brine from the bag if needed. Let the cucumbers ferment until they become an even olive green color, about 2½ to 3 weeks. Taste a pickle. If it has good dill flavor and a sour taste, they're done. If you want more sourness, allow them to continue fermenting, but no longer than 3 weeks. Pour off the brine into the stainless steel or other nonreactive pot through several layers of cheesecloth to remove the solids and impurities. For immediate consumption, up to 6 to 8 weeks, store the pickles in the refrigerator in jars topped up with the brine. For long-term storage, you'll have to can your pickles.

Gingered Carrots

There's something about the flavor of ginger that augments the flavor of garden-fresh carrots. If you're not growing your own, look for carrots with their tops on at the market. If the tops appear bright green, aromatic, and fresh, the carrots will be, too. The fermentation period helps these two disparate-but-symbiotic flavors to meld and mellow.

*MAKES 1 QUART

Ingredients

    4 cups tightly packed grated carrots
    1 tablespoon peeled, grated fresh ginger
    3 teaspoons sea salt or pickling salt

Method

✳ IN A LARGE BOWL, mix the carrots, ginger, and salt together and set the bowl aside for 30 minutes. Using a wooden pounder or potato masher, pound the carrot mixture for 5 minutes so the vegetables release their juices. Place the contents of the bowl in a quart canning jar and press down firmly so the carrots are covered by juice. Add filtered water to just cover the carrots as needed. Leave 1 inch of headspace between the top of the juice and the top of the jar. Place a single sheet of paper towel over the jar and screw on the band that holds the jar's metal lid. Set the jar on a warm kitchen counter for 5 days. Check the jar each day and remove any scum that rises; keeping the vegetables submerged will prevent any spoilage. Then cover the jar with a metal jar lid before placing it in the refrigerator, where it will keep for 3 to 4 weeks.

Sauerkraut

Cabbage, like many of the cole crops (its cruciferous relatives in the plant world), grows well in cool weather, which is why it was grown extensively across Northern Europe and the northern tier of the United States in the seventeenth through nineteenth centuries, before refrigeration. Winter closes in fast in these cold regions, and hard freezes would destroy the cabbage that provided farmers with greens and vitamin C during the long, freezing months.

And so these farmers learned to do a simple trick—brine their cabbage until the vegetable was fermented and stabilized, whereupon the cabbage would last just fine in cold storage during the winter. When some was needed for the table, it was just fished out of the crock and the lid replaced. As we now know, cabbage is a wonderfully nutritious food, providing vitamin C and other essential nutrients, protecting the human body against diseases such as cancer, and the Lactobacilli *that colonize the sauerkraut release bound-up nutritive factors in the cabbage—sauerkraut contains twenty times more bioavailable vitamin C than raw cabbage—and for the human gut.*

*MAKES 4 QUARTS

Ingredients

5 pounds (2 or 3 heads) cabbage

3 tablespoons sea salt or pickling salt (non-iodized)

Method

✳ REMOVE JUST THE outer leaves of the cabbage and slice the heads in half through the core. Using a sharp knife or a mandolin, slice the cabbage into shreds and discard the core when finished. You can also remove the cores before slicing. Place the shredded cabbage in a large bowl. As you add handfuls, sprinkle the cabbage with a little salt. When all of the cabbage is shredded and in the bowl, add the remaining salt.

✳ USING YOUR HANDS, toss, squeeze, pound, crunch, and massage the cabbage for about 10 minutes, until the shreds grow limp and the cabbage juices start to run. As the cabbage turns limp and juicy, use a wooden mallet or pounder to finish the cabbage for the last 3 or 4 minutes.

✳ PLACE THE CABBAGE IN a small ceramic crock or widemouthed 1-gallon glass jar. Place a plate that fits in the crock or jar on top of the cabbage and press down hard to work any air bubbles out of the cabbage. Weigh down the plate with a gallon jug of water or with a zip-top freezer bag filled with brine. Place the bag unsealed on the plate with the seal up so it spreads to cover the plate and any juice showing between the plate and crock. Then seal it. The juice should completely cover the cabbage. If there's not enough juice to cover the cabbage, put a little extra brine in the crock or jar until the cabbage is entirely under the liquid.

✳ COVER THE CROCK OR JAR with a clean dish towel held in place with a rubber band and store it in a place that ideally is between 70°F and 75°F. Check the crock or jar after a couple of days and every few days after that. It will start to ferment (bubble) after a few days. If you see any mold growing on the surface of the liquid, remove the weight bag or jug and the plate and skim off as much as you can. Don't worry, the sauerkraut is safe as long as it's submerged under the brine. Just get as much scum or mold off the liquid as you can and replace the plate, weight, and towel. The kraut will improve in flavor over the next month or two. If you find it exactly at the place you like it, pack the kraut into canning jars with brine to cover and store them in the refrigerator, where it will last for several months as long as the kraut is covered with brine. Rinse the kraut to remove salt before serving if you wish.

German Apples and Kraut

*MAKES 2 QUARTS

Ingredients

1 medium head ball cabbage, shredded
1 teaspoon sea salt or pickling salt (non-iodized)
2 firm apples, peeled, cored, and shredded
1 teaspoon grated fresh ginger

Method

✳ IN A LARGE BOWL, combine the cabbage and salt. Work the salt through the cabbage, massaging the shreds for 5 to 10 minutes, until the cabbage juice runs. Add the shredded apples and ginger and then massage again for a minute to incorporate. Pack the kraut into a small crock or glass or ceramic bowl and place a plate on the top. Set a quart canning jar filled with water and with its lid screwed on as a weight on the plate. If there's not enough juice to cover the cabbage, add just a bit of water until the cabbage is covered. Cover the crock or bowl with a clean dish towel.

✳ PLACE THE KRAUT CONTAINER in a warm place—70°F to 75°F is ideal—for a week, checking daily to skim any foam from the top and removing the weight and plate and stirring the kraut 2 or 3 times during the week. Strain the kraut, reserving the juices in a bowl. Pack the apples and sauerkraut into quart glass canning jars, adding enough of the reserved juice to keep the kraut wet, and store in the refrigerator. The kraut lasts for 2 or 3 weeks.

Index

ALSO BY ROBYNNE CHUTKAN, M.D.

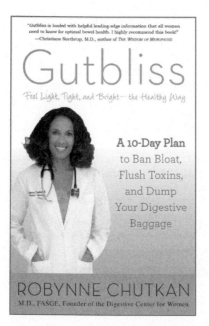

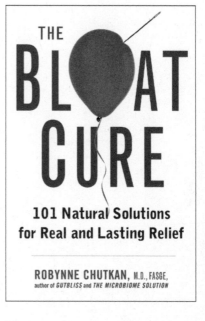

A complete guide to good gastrointestinal health for women, with a ten-day digestive tune-up.

The must-have A to Z manual to banish your bloat for good.

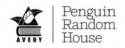